FIT AND FLEXIBLE AT 50

FIT AND FLEXIBLE AT 50

How I Lost 50 pounds
at 50 Years Old
and Became The
Most Flexible
I've Ever Been

STEVE MONROE

This book is intended for informational and educational purposes only and is based on the personal experiences of the author. It is not intended as medical advice, nutritional advice, or a substitute for professional guidance.

The author is not a physician, dietitian, or licensed medical professional. Always consult with a qualified healthcare provider before making changes to your diet, exercise routine, or lifestyle, especially if you have a medical condition or health concerns.

Individual results may vary.
What worked for the author may not work the same way for everyone.

Copyright © 2026 Steve Monroe

All rights reserved. No part of this book may be reproduced, distributed, or transmitted in any form or by any means, including photocopying, recording, or other electronic or mechanical methods, without the prior written permission of the author, except in the case of brief quotations embodied in critical reviews and certain other non-commercial uses permitted by copyright law.

Printed in the United States of America

Published by Monroe Media Group, LLC

Library of Congress Cataloging-in-Publication Data is on file with the publisher:
ISBN 979-8-9945358-5-1

For my parents,
thank you for the foundation of love,
and embracing creativity,
and encouraging curiosity,
and enforcing the beliefs
that made everything possible,
and,
and,
and.

CONTENTS

Introduction

PART I — The Wake-Up

Chapter 1 — The Summer My Name Mattered	3
Studying Skills	8
Coach Pat Alexander	9
Chapter 2 — Fat-Faced Fortune	11
The "Dirty Windshield"	12
The Wheel of Fortune	14
Chapter 3 — The Pandemic Pivot	15
Three Phases of Diet	16
The Exercise Shift	17

PART II — The Build

Chapter 4 — Fit and Flexible Starter Meals	21
Essential Kitchen Tools	21
Let's Talk About Cow's Milk	24
Chapter 5 — Get Ready to Get Ready	55
The Reality Check Nobody Warns You About	55
Set Your Agreements With Yourself	61
Earn Your Body's Trust	69
Chapter 6 — The Seven-Day Master Cleanse (The Reset)	71
What the Master Cleanse Actually Is	71
Why It Works	72
The Emotional & Physical Timeline	76

The Organic Vegetable Soup	80
Chapter 7 — 90-Day Game Plan: Meals, Movement, Momentum	83
Weekly Meal Templates	85
How Movement Anchors Identity	88
Acting Like the Person You Want to Become	92
Chapter 8 — The Fit & Flexible Recipe Library	95
The Meals That Did the Heavy Lifting	95
Recipe Library	98

PART III — The Shift

Chapter 9 — Mindset: The Identity Shift	165
It Showed Up as Silence	165
Chapter 10 — MicroStrategies That Shaped My Journey	171
Mini-Losses Don't Matter — Repetition Does	173
Prep Today for Tomorrow	174
Fast-Food Pivots (Survival Without Shame)	179
Chapter 11 — Results: Fit and Flexible at 50	182
The Feeling (What Changed Internally)	185
The Identity Shift Made Visible	186
Why This Is Sustainable	190
Chapter 12 — Now It's Your Turn	192
Start Where You Are	195
What Actually Matters	196
The Next Right Move	197
Epilogue — Five Years Later	199
Acknowledgments & Influences	203

INTRODUCTION

I Am Not a Doctor (And That's Kind of the Point)

Let's get something out of the way right now.

I am not a doctor, but I have played one on T.V. Well, Intern really. I am one of the faces in the OR with McDreamy in season two of Grey's Anatomy. Dr. Shepard flawlessly performs brain surgery while finding out that all of our lives are at risk from a live ordinance inside of a patient in the room next us. The tension was thick.

Okay, while that was a true story but, back to reality. I am not a nutritionist. I do not have a lab coat, a prescription pad, or a framed degree hanging on the wall behind me.

I will never try to explain to you the metabolic pathways using words that end in –ology. **I am not qualified to write that book.**

I am only qualified to write a book about my story. My story is about a gradual drift. A steady relationship with comfort food, date night at local restaurants, travel, late nights, and working in an industry built around sitting, flying, and poor eating choices. Life choices eventually added up. There was no crisis, no diet-program hopping—just the compound effect of small lifestyle adjustments that didn't seem to matter until they did.

This book is not written from theory. It's written from experience.

My Credentials Are Mileage

My background isn't in medicine. It's in life, work, travel, late nights, early mornings, airports, hotel gyms, country clubs, comedy clubs, and more than a few "I'll start Monday" Mondays.

For 25 years, I've made a living in and around the entertainment industry. That means long hours, unpredictable schedules, extended road trips, social meals, late dinners, drinks that "come with the room," and food that exists because it's convenient—not because it's good for you.

It also means something else that matters more than people realize: I had to function.

I couldn't disappear into a monk-like routine. I couldn't meal prep like I was training for a bodybuilding show. I couldn't shut down my calendar for six months and "focus on my health."

Whatever I did had to work inside a real adult life.

About the Medical Stuff (Because Yes, We're Going There)

When this book references physiology, digestion, inflammation, insulin, or recovery, it's not to play doctor. It's to give you context, not commands.

I respect medicine deeply. My mother was a nurse for over 40 years. Highly trained doctors saved my father's life while he was suffering from a leaking brain aneurysm. Emergency medicine, diagnostics, and surgery are miracles of modern civilization.

But this book is not about treating disease.

It's about eating better than you were, moving more than you did, reducing inflammation and fatigue, and creating momentum instead of restarting every January.

This is **lifestyle engineering**, not medical treatment.

If you have medical conditions, medications, or specific health concerns, you should absolutely involve your doctor. This book is not a replacement for professional care.

It's a framework for people who are tired of knowing what they *should* do—and want something they can actually sustain.

Why You Can Trust This Anyway

You don't need a doctor to tell you:

- Ultra-processed food makes you feel worse
- Consistent movement beats sporadic hero workouts
- Structure reduces decision fatigue
- Walking works
- Sleep matters
- Less chaos equals better results

What you need is someone who tested these truths in the middle of a busy, imperfect life—and shows you how to apply them without burning everything down.

That's what I'm offering.

Not authority. Not perfection. **Proof of work.**

The Promise of This Book

- I will never ask you to do something I didn't do.
- I will never recommend something I couldn't sustain.
- I will never pretend this is magic.

What I will give you is a system that respects your life, meets you where you are, leaves room for humor, mistakes, and momentum, and actually works if you work it.

No white coat required.

PART I — The Wake-Up
Where awareness begins the change.

CHAPTER ONE

The Summer My Name Mattered

Before I ever understood nutrition, fitness, or consistency, I accidentally learned something far more important.

Like more than half of American kids, I come from a broken family. My parents separated before I was three. I lived with my single mom until I was ten, and then with my single dad through the end of high school. Both of my parents are absolute angels—strong, loving, deeply influential people in my life—and I wouldn't be who I am without either of them. At the same time, they each had their own struggles. What we didn't have was stability. If you grew up with it, you know exactly what I mean. Same house. Same street. Same elementary school. Same junior high. Same high school. Same friends. Groundhog Day, over and over again. Yeah… that was definitely not me.

I attended eight elementary schools and three junior high schools before finally settling into one high school after eighth grade. Constantly being the new kid in a room full of strangers left me disconnected and disoriented. After a while, it felt pointless to invest. Homework didn't matter. Studying didn't matter. Responsibility and accountability didn't matter.

When I was twelve years old, Halloween was getting close, and I was obsessed with Kiss—especially Gene Simmons. The makeup. The blood. The fire. I didn't just like the band; I was fascinated by the character. I wanted to *Rock and Roll All Night and Party Every Day!*

The problem was, I was twelve and had no money. So, I created a plan. A flawless plan really. My local candy bar spot, Kirk's Drugs, was only three blocks away. I knew exactly where they kept the seasonal Halloween makeup packages. I knew what aisle they were on. I knew exactly what I was going to do. I visualized the entire route. I was confident!

I walked into the store, went straight to the aisle, and most definitely did not look both ways. I grabbed a Halloween makeup kit, slid it under my shirt, down my pants, and walked out.

I didn't get far.

A clerk came out the door behind me and said, "Young man, one of the other shoppers said they saw you put something in your pants. Is that true?"

A seasoned criminal would have held a poker face, given a convincing denial, probably said something dismissive, maybe even combative. I never got that far in my "flawless plan." In that moment, I remembered something my father always said, "Kid, you're going to fuck up in life. Never lie about it. Don't be a fuck up AND a liar."

So, I said what came naturally, "Yes."

I was taken into the office to wait for the police. Kirk, the owner, sat across his desk from me. He gently shook his head, and said, "Your father's not going to be very proud of this."

I looked up at him and said, "You know my dad?"

He nodded. "Oh yeah. I know your dad."

And that's when I realized I wasn't just in trouble—I was known.

I was given a court date. Because it was my first offense, I got a slap on the wrist. A warning. I walked away.

Another big lesson that I took from that experience is that nothing screams masculinity like being a twelve-year-old boy getting caught stealing makeup.

Fast forward to the end of seventh grade. We had moved to the other side of Lacey, Washington. Like most kids growing up there, we played capture the flag in the forest—sometimes late into the night. One night around 12:30 a.m., my friend Arthur and I were walking home when we heard banging coming from Nisqually Middle School.

Like young boys do, we went to investigate. Two eighth graders had broken into the janitor's closet from the roof. One of them tossed me a pencil sharpener. I put it in my backpack. We left the scene. Arthur went home. I went my way.

Once again, I didn't get far.

A sheriff picked me up on the side of the road and drove me through the school so I could see the chaos—spray paint, vandalism, angry messages toward teachers. I remember sitting in the back of the police car crying, pleading, "I don't want to be blamed for all of this."

By 1:30 a.m. the Sheriff had awakened Arthur's family. My accomplice revealed. My story validated. At 2:30 in the morning, the police knocked on my door and delivered his juvenile delinquent son back to a surprised and embarrassed father. I will not pollute this chapter with the language my father used to express his anger and frustration.

The following Monday, Arthur and I sat in the principal's office, flipped through the yearbook, and identified the two boys responsible—I've chosen not to write the names to protect the guilty.

Even so, I was cited for trespassing and possession of stolen property. This time, I didn't walk away. About six months later, I was sentenced to 200 hours of community service.

Before my sentencing, during the summer before Eight grade, we moved again. This time to the other side of the county to Tumwater. This is where I got lucky.

Unlike many of the other young criminals, I did not have to join a freeway clean up crew dressed in a bright jumpsuit and pick up trash. Thankfully, one of my dad's close friends worked at the Tumwater Fire

Station, on the corner of Capitol Boulevard and Israel Road, so that's where I "served my hard time."

After school, day after day, I got to walk the Dalmatian, wash fire trucks, sweep floors, organize gear, and clean the station. And I was surrounded by men. I wasn't around any men—I was around THE men. The first responders. Men of brotherhood. Men of accountability. Men of bravery.

About two and a half weeks into gathering my hours, I asked my dad's friend if he could sign my paper for the day. He told me, "The captain wants to sign them today."

The captain asked me to walk with him around the station so he could see the work I'd been doing. I was super excited. Until I wasn't.

We stopped near one of the fire trucks. He pointed underneath and barked, "What the fuck is this?"

I had never been spoken to like that by someone I had just met. "It's… it's dust," I stuttered.

"You can't sweep under fire trucks," he said.

I stumbled on my words once again, "The broom doesn't reach, sir."

He looked at me and said, "You don't think we have keys? You don't think we'd move the truck if you asked so you could do a hundred percent of the job you were given?"

My right knee began to shake. "I'm sorry, sir."

"Sorry doesn't cut it in my firehouse," he said.
 "Sorry costs people their lives."

Without another word, he walked away, and I realized I was supposed to follow him. He went over to the side of another fire truck that I had just washed. He pointed at the side of it.

"What the fuck are those?"

I stood there staring at several missed spots—those diamond-shaped patches you leave when your hand doesn't quite reach every inch.

Looking at his feet, I said, "Um, spots, sir."

"Look at me please." He firmly asked, "Do you expect my guys to risk their lives in a fire truck that looks like the fucking dog?"

The Dalmatian reference almost landed as a joke. Almost.

Then, the captain became calm. He knelt down on one knee, held me squarely by the shoulders, took a deep breath, looked me right in the eyes, stared into my soul, and said the sentence that changed my young life.

"Steve, you are at an age where you must realize that everything you do has your name on it. You are the only one who can decide how you want to be remembered."

"I want you to think about what I just told you while you finish the job," he said. Because if you are not willing to give one hundred percent alongside the men who are risking their lives for your town, you are no longer welcome in my fire station."

And he walked away.

He gave me an extra hour—with no credit—to redo the work.

During that hour, there was a massive shift. I became a better son. I became a better student. I became a better athlete. I became more than a kid who did things halfway.

Looking back, I realize that the captain was not just teaching me discipline. The captain treated me like someone who will matters.

Studying Skills

However, that shift didn't erase the damage that had already been done. Years of bouncing from school to school had caught up with me. By the end of eighth grade, I had still failed eight classes. Not assignments. Classes. Nearly a third of my schedule. Because I had started school a year early, I was already younger than everyone else—and now I was staring down the real possibility of being held back.

When the high school counselors sat me down, they made it clear this wasn't a negotiation. I could move forward into ninth grade with my friends, but only under two conditions: they would choose my classes, and one of those classes had to be Study Skills.

To get to the fire station, I had to walk. I would leave the junior high, head down Israel Road, walk over the freeway overpass, pass right by the high school, and keep going until I reached the fire station on the corner of Capitol Boulevard. I made that walk every day for weeks. At first, walking past the high school felt exciting. A fresh start. Freedom.

Somewhere between finishing my community service hours and sitting in the principal's office, I went from assuming I'd be going there… to not being sure I'd be allowed to. So every afternoon, I walked past the future I thought I was headed toward, not knowing if I'd already disqualified myself from it. That uncertainty stayed with me longer than the punishment ever did.

At that point, moving forward wasn't about choice anymore, it was about permission.

If I hadn't learned from the fire captain that my name mattered—that effort mattered—I would have walked into Study Skills the same way I walked into every other class before it. Detached. Indifferent. Just passing time until my next move. When the counselor told me I could move forward into high school under two conditions—that they would choose my classes, and that one of them had to be Study Skills—I didn't argue. A year earlier, I would have nodded and said, "Sure. Whatever."

And I would have meant it.

But that summer changed something. I had already learned what it felt like to put my name on something and be held to it. So when I walked into Pat Alexander's classroom, I wasn't motivated. I was ready.

Coach Pat Alexander

Coach Pat Alexander wasn't the kind of teacher you forgot. This teacher was one of the Assistant football coaches. He was also one of the wrestling coaches. I didn't play football or wrestle—baseball and soccer were my jam—but he carried himself with the same presence I had just experienced at the fire station. Standards mattered to him. But what he taught us in Study Skills had very little to do with homework. That class wasn't about color-coding notebooks or cramming for tests. It was about how your mind works.

Coach Alexander was the man who taught the football team to G.A.T.A. (Get After Their Ass). Pat Alexander was also the man who preached, "If it is to be, it is up to me." Pat also wasn't afraid to tell those he cared about, "I love you a whole skyful."

Pat Alexander taught us the difference between the conscious mind—the voice you hear all day long—and the subconscious mind, which he described as the most powerful supercomputer in the world. Your subconscious listens to your conscious voice. It takes notes. And then it works around the clock to make what you say true.

If you say: "I can't remember names," your subconscious doesn't spend the night trying to help you remember names better. It accepts that statement as an instruction.

If you say: "I'm bad at math," it starts looking for proof.

If you say: "I'm terrible at taking tests," your subconscious mind builds a system that makes sure you are.

What you speak, you slowly become. Yes, it sounds redundant. If you had to reread it, I get it. That's because it's uncomfortable to realize how much power our own inner voice has had this whole time.

That first trimester of freshman year, I failed algebra. I picked up a few C's. I got an A in P.E., obviously. But I also got an A in Study Skills. Coach Alexander required something very powerful from all of us. When you entered his class. You had to be doing "GREAT!"

He would ask every day, "How are you doing Steve?"

There was only one answer. "GREAT!" It was non-negotiable! That simple, but effective requirement mattered more than it sounds. Because something had shifted. For the first time, I wasn't just being held accountable for effort—I was learning how to hold myself accountable internally. I had learned from the fire captain that sorry doesn't cut it. Coach Pat Alexander taught me that the words you privately speak to yourself decide whether effort has the foundation to grow.

From that point forward, I never failed another class. As and Bs for the rest of my high school career. In the end, I actually graduated with honors. Not because I suddenly became smarter, but because I had learned two things, in the same season of my life, that finally worked together.

The Fire Captain taught me how I see my name matters. Coach Pat Alexander taught me how I hear my voice matters.

Long before I ever changed my body, I was learning how change actually works.

CHAPTER TWO

Fat-Faced Fortune

I never thought I'd be writing about losing weight. Honestly, growing up, I was the exact opposite of the "before" picture. I was a lean kid. Nobody ever looked at me and thought, "Yeah, this guy could hold something down." No, I was the one who got asked to crawl under the house and fix the cables. I was the designated tight-space specialist.

Throughout high school and college I was always active in sports. For most of my life, my metabolism had my back. Friends and family warned me. "Wait until your 30s, Steve—your metabolism will catch up to you."

Nope. Made it through.

"Well, it'll get you in your 40s."

Nope again. Still cruising, still lean.

I figured maybe I was immune. Maybe I was one of the chosen few. The guy who could slam a burrito at 2 a.m. and wake up with abs. But as it turns out, God wasn't giving me a pass—He was just letting me build up a tab.

The Flight Industry Life

What finally did me in wasn't age—it was lifestyle. I got into a comfortable domestic relationship, which shifted my eating and exercise habits. And then came the flight industry.

If you know anything about that life, it's a fitness graveyard. Constant body compression from takeoffs and landings. Hydration? Usually adult beverages at midnight. Meals? Airport food. High carb, high fat, high regret. Exercise? The only thing I was lifting was my feet off the floor and onto the bed.

And the snacks. Oh, the snacks.

Fritos by the bag, except they disguised themselves in those little 100-calorie packs. One bag didn't seem bad—until you flew four legs in a day. Oreos came in neat little four-packs, easy to justify, until you grabbed two of them for the hotel room.

And my biggest nemesis? Dr. Pepper. Oh, I loved Dr. Pepper. Who am I kidding—love Dr. Pepper. Sometimes I would choose a fast-food restaurant based on whether or not they had it. Actually, let's be honest: all the time. Free Dr. Pepper on every flight didn't help. Half a can here, a full can there. The compound effect of sugar is inevitable.

And the worst part? We had a secret compartment in the galley where we could stash as many snacks as we wanted. A snack speakeasy. Except instead of whiskey, we were bootlegging Fritos and Oreos.

The Dirty Windshield

The weight didn't slam into me all at once—it snuck in. A pound here, a pound there. Like windshield wipers slowly wearing down, you don't notice how bad they are until you put new ones on and—oh my God—I can see.

I had experienced the taste of eating clean and working out earlier in my flight career with the Body Beast program, and it was incredible. But then came a five-day trip to Puerto Vallarta. Margaritas. Chips. Salsa. Guacamole. Paradise, right? Except I fell hard off the wagon—and never got back on.

That's when the slow-motion slide started. Airport food, adult beverages, late-night flights, missed workouts. The warning signs were there. My scale creeped past 182—the heaviest I'd ever been since a snowboarding accident in 1999. My flexibility disappearing—I couldn't even touch my toes anymore. And the big one: when I got refitted for a new uniform, the tailor told me my waist was 36. I thought, "There's definitely something wrong with that tape measure." Warning signs.

Taste and Toss

Did I listen? Kind of. I adopted a weird little mental philosophy to trick myself. Instead of devouring an entire bag of Fritos, I'd open it, throw three or four chips in my mouth, and while chewing that salty, crunchy perfection, I'd dump the rest straight into the trash. Same with Oreos: I'd open a four-pack, take one bite—just half an Oreo—and toss the rest.

Sounds wasteful, right? But it worked. I got the flavor, the salty-sweet gratification, without the crash of overindulgence. Sometimes the difference between staying on track and falling off the rails is learning how to taste without needing to finish.

Did it solve the problem? No. But it was my first attempt at wrestling with it.

The Dad Bod Without the Dad Card

By the time my weight climbed over 190, then 200, golf was my main hobby. But I wasn't walking the course. I was riding in a cart, and the heaviest thing I was lifting was the cooler lid. Then came the audition that changed everything.

Somehow, I landed one of the rarest tickets in America: Wheel of Fortune. With just barely over 7,000 shows and three contestants per episode, less than 22,000 people have ever made it onto that stage. And I was one of them.

And here's the part I hate to admit: I knew I was overweight. Weeks before the big day, I ordered a men's Spanx. A body-trimming tank top. I was trying to camouflage my dad bod—even though everybody knew I wasn't a dad. I wore it. But no amount of Lycra was going to save me from what came next.

The Wheel of Fortune

On March 13th, 2020—yes, Friday the 13th—I stepped on the Wheel of Fortune stage. I spun. I solved it. I even flirted dangerously close to the million-dollar wedge. And then I landed on the tiniest bankrupt sliver, sandwiched between two million-dollar slices. My life in one spin: almost major success, but just enough space for disaster. Just kidding, that is not a metaphor for my life.

Off camera Pat tried to console me, "Do you know how accurate you have to be to hit that space?"

"Thanks Pat!"

A few weeks later came the real hit, the studio sent me my official contestant headshot. The headshot hit harder than the wheel ever could.

That was my bankrupt moment. For the first time in my life, I looked at a photo and thought, "Oh my God… I have a fat face."

And to top it all off, the pandemic was now in full swing.

Friday the 13th hit the world extremely hard.

That's when everything changed.

CHAPTER THREE
The Pandemic Pivot

When I got that Wheel of Fortune headshot back, I couldn't unsee it. My fat face stared back at me like an unwelcome houseguest who'd moved in without permission. Then the pandemic shut the world down, and suddenly there was no travel, no airport food, no galley snack speakeasy, no free-flowing Dr. Pepper on every flight.

It was absolute timing. I had to face myself. No distractions. And it came down to the oldest equation in the book: diet and exercise.

The Diet Shift

During the first few weeks of the global shutdown, I leaned the wrong way. With flights grounded and restaurants closed, I started cooking at home... and I was pumped about it. If I was going to cook, I was going to go big. Think decadent meals dripping with fat. Brownie-cookie combo desserts, and ice cream on the side. Quarantine was basically my audition for Top Chef: Dessert Island... except there was no one else there to vote me off.

But then I stumbled on a book that changed everything: Wheat Belly by Dr. William Davis.

That book was a gut punch—literally. It talked about visceral fat, the fat you don't just see on the surface, but that builds around your organs. And I thought, Oh no, that's me. I had a dad bod... without being a dad. The book explained how our modern grains had evolved, how our bodies respond, and why that stubborn layer of fat builds up. It didn't just alarm me—it made sense. So I decided to try it.

I started pulling recipes from the Wheat Belly book, saving them in Recipe Keeper, and watching YouTube cooking tutorials like my life depended on it. For the first time in my life, I wasn't just reheating—I was cooking. And you know what? I actually enjoyed it. Trader Joe's chocolate peanut butter protein bars became my Oreo replacement. I had tasty meals, better snacks, and for once, I was excited about what I was eating.

Three Phases of Diet

Looking back, my transition happened in three clear phases:

Three Weeks of Learning Cooking with YouTube. Experimenting with recipes. Building my menus. (And failing a few times. Note to self: coconut flour is not the same as wheat flour, no matter how hopeful you are.)

Ten Days of the Master Cleanse This one needed strategy. I had tried it once before during P90X and failed miserably. So this time, I found a partner. Someone else who had failed once, just like me. We became Cleanse buddies. For seven full days we stuck it out, then properly exited the Cleanse over the next two days. It was brutal, but it reset my system.

Four Months of Execution Post-Cleanse, I had the knowledge, the skills, the menus, and the recipes. All I had to do was keep making the good foods and keep choosing the good snacks. That's it.

The result? In those five months I dropped 50 pounds. From 206 pounds down to 156, with a 31-inch waist—the same waistline I had in high school.

The Exercise Shift

Exercise during the pandemic wasn't complicated—it was stripped down to two things: stretching and walking. Gyms were closed. Group sports were out. But golf survived.

I don't like walking or running just for the sake of it. I need to do something. Golf gave me the best excuse. So, I quit riding in carts. I bought a push cart and started walking the course.

Nine holes = 2.5+ miles.

Eighteen holes = up to 8 miles.

No beers, no alcohol on the course this time. I was taking my body and my game more seriously, and those steps added up.

The second "Athletic" adjustment I made was, I added P90X Stretch to my mornings — 45 minutes of yoga-inspired stretching, keeping my body flexible, my joints mobile, and my head clear.

That was it. Stretching and walking. The most underrated workout combo on Earth.

Keep It Simple

You don't need a complicated workout plan or a $2,000 home gym to get results. I am also sure you don't have a set of P90X CDs sitting in a drawer like I did. That's okay! I have since upgraded to using an app known mainly for their cycling workouts. Most yoga inspired apps have several great 30-45 minute, easy flow sessions, to get even the most basic beginner making progress towards your goals.

Stretching + walking, paired with a consistent eating strategy, can move the needle more than you think. Start where you are, with what you can do, and let consistency do the heavy lifting.

PART II — The Build
Where preparation strengthens willpower

CHAPTER FOUR
Fit & Flexible Starter Meals

Before we can talk about meals, menus, or mastering nutrition, we need to talk about one simple truth: Your kitchen is either your greatest ally… or a storage room where takeout containers go to die.

When I started this journey, I wasn't trying to become a chef. I was just trying to survive. But it didn't take long to realize that a few essential tools could transform cooking from a chore into something enjoyable — even exciting. So before we dive into breakfasts that fuel your mornings and dinners that build your body, let's talk about the gear.

ESSENTIAL KITCHEN TOOLS:

1. The Magic Bullet (a tiny blender with heroic energy)
2. The Instant Pot (so good, I bought two)
3. The Wok (my culinary lightsaber)
4. The Air Fryer (comfort food without the guilt)

The Magic Bullet

It was small, fast, and didn't require a 12-step cleaning ritual. If your goal is consistency — and trust me, consistency is everything — you need a blender you'll actually use.

- Smoothies
- Protein shakes
- Mixing ingredients
- Grinding seeds
- Blending sauces

The Instant Pot - The Swiss Army knife for the kitchen

I didn't just fall in love with the Instant Pot — I committed to it!! Why? Because it can do everything! The Instant Pot absolutely elevated my kitchen game!. It made everything so fast, and easy.

- Rice cooker
- Crockpot
- Steamer
- Pressure cooker
- Pasta maker
- Soup master
- Meal maker
- Vegetable whisperer
- Chicken tender superstar

Once I realized I could make perfect rice in one Instant Pot while perfect chicken cooked in the other — I understood enlightenment. It also cleans easily. The Instant Pot fits my lifestyle effortlessly.

The first meal I made in the Instant Pot was so good, I bought another one. One for the main dish, one for the sides. The most fun is trying to guess the right timing and have the main dish and the side dish finish at the same time!

Who doesn't like finishing at the same time?

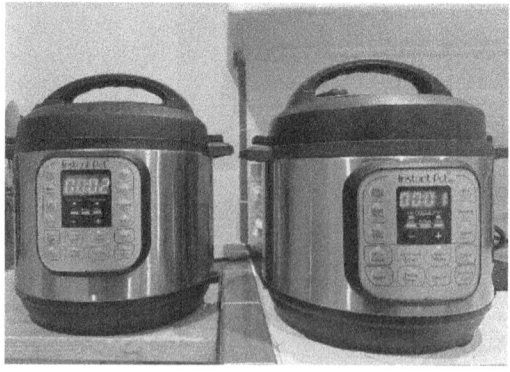

Two Pots. One Goal

The Wok - My Culinary Lightsaber

If the Instant Pot is John Rambo's Swiss Army knife of the kitchen, the Wok is Luke Skywalker's lightsaber.

It transforms vegetables. It brings proteins to life. It delivers flavor like you trained under a Michelin-star Jedi Master. I love the Wok because:

- It cooks large volumes easily
- It caramelizes vegetables beautifully
- It builds layers of flavor
- It transitions perfectly when adding a protein

And best of all? Next morning, you toss in Wok leftovers + a couple of eggs, and BOOM: Bonus Breakfast. One of the greatest hacks of this entire journey.

The Air Fryer

An air fryer earns its place because it delivers crisp, satisfying food with less oil and keeps meals enjoyable when reheated, which makes consistency far easier to maintain.

- Creates crisp texture without deep frying
- Uses far less oil than traditional methods
- Reheats food evenly while preserving texture
- Keeps leftovers tasting intentional, not compromised
- You can reheat almost anything in here

When food still tastes good the second time around, sticking to a smart, structured eating plan stops feeling like work and starts feeling automatic. Now that we have the tools, let's put them to use…

Let's talk about Cow's milk.

As Meghan Trainor says: "It's all about that base, 'bout that base."
That's one thing I learned early on. Every protein shake is only as good as its base.

So, before we talk about protein powder, fruit, or any add-ins, we need to talk about something far more important:

Cow's milk!

There it is! I said it!

When I was a kid, I loved milk. I couldn't wait to finish my cereal so I could drink that glorious, sugary milk at the bottom of the bowl. While some kids wanted just barely enough milk to choke down their cereal, I was filling my bowl until the cereal would threaten mutiny and fall over the edge of the bowl. I had Milk with a lunchtime sandwich. Milk with dinner. And eventually, milk in my protein shakes. Milk was practically a food group in my life.

So, what changed? About twenty years ago, I read an article in a fitness magazine that stopped me mid-sip. It broke down two simple, undeniable facts:

Humans are the only mammals who drink milk after the weaning process.

All other mammals switch to nature's elixir… water. We like to think of ourselves as the most evolved creatures on the planet, but apparently we're the only ones who never got the memo: milk is NOT a lifelong beverage.

We are the only mammals who drink another mammal's milk.

A goat has never — in the history of the world — knocked on the side of a cow and said, "Hey, can I borrow your udder and grab a glass for the kids?"

Then the article explained:

Milk has to be cooked to be digestible for humans.

It turns sour if not consumed quickly.

Honestly, how many times have you opened the lid of a milk jug and taken a cautious sniff before deciding whether to risk it? Why do we do that to ourselves?

And just like that, everything clicked. That was the last day cow's milk ever crossed my lips.

What is my base of choice? Unsweetened vanilla almond milk. Creamy. Smooth. Perfect for blending. And it made my shakes taste closer to dessert instead and nothing like punishment.

So, here we go…

Breakfast #1 - Super Fruit Protein Shake

This is the quick morning shake that jump-started my transformation. It is the ultimate no-excuses breakfast for mornings when time is tight but standards are still high. It's built to deliver solid protein, fiber, and nutrients in one smooth move, without leaving you hungry an hour later. Think of it as a reliable bridge between "I should eat" and "I have five minutes."

Serving Size: 1 serving

INGREDIENTS

- 8-10 oz unsweetened vanilla almond milk
- 1½ scoops protein powder
- ½ frozen banana
- 1 tablespoon peanut butter
- ¼-⅓ cup frozen mixed berries (raspberry/blackberry/blueberry combo)
- ¼ cup frozen spinach
- 1 tablespoon chia seeds
- 1 teaspoon creatine

NUTRITION (Per Serving)

Calories: ~448
Protein: ~44 g
Carbohydrates: ~34 g
Fiber: ~9 g
Sugars: ~13 g
Fat: ~17 g
Saturated Fat: ~4-5 g
Sodium: ~470 mg

HOW TO MAKE IT:

1. Add almond milk to the Magic Bullet.
2. Toss in frozen banana.
3. Add peanut butter.
4. Add protein powder, creatine, and chia seeds.
5. Add berries.
6. Blend until smooth.

Refreshing Fruit Variation

It's built to deliver solid protein, fiber, and nutrients in one smooth move, without leaving you hungry an hour later. The pineapple–mango version keeps things light and refreshing.

INGREDIENTS

- Swap berries for: Frozen pineapple, frozen mango, or both

NUTRITION (Per Serving)

Calories: ~452
Protein: ~44 g
Carbohydrates: ~36 g
Fiber: ~6 g
Sugars: ~19 g
Fat: ~17 g
Saturated Fat: ~4-5 g
Sodium: ~470 mg

Chocolate Peanut Butter Option

The chocolate peanut butter option tastes like a Chocolate Peanut Butter cup that somehow still supports your goals.

INGREDIENTS

- 8-10 oz almond milk
- 1½ scoops chocolate protein powder
- ½ frozen banana
- 1 tablespoon peanut butter
- 1 teaspoon creatine

NUTRITION (Per Serving)

Calories: ~428
Protein: ~44 g Fiber: ~4 g
Sugars: ~12 g
Fat: ~15 g
Saturated Fat: ~4 g
Sodium: ~320 mg

Breakfast #2 - Turkey Bacon, Eggs & Spinach Scramble

This is a high-protein, low-nonsense breakfast that hits hard without feeling heavy. It's fast, filling, and flexible — perfect for mornings when you want real food, real energy, and zero decision fatigue. If you're training, traveling, or just trying to stay on track, this scramble does the job.

Serving Size: 1 serving

INGREDIENTS

- 6 slices turkey bacon
- 2 large whole eggs
- 4 additional large egg whites
- ⅓ cup spinach
- 4 cherry tomatoes, halved
- ¼ cup reduced-fat pepper jack cheese
- 1 teaspoon olive oil
- Salt, to taste
- Pepper, to taste

HOW TO MAKE IT:

1. Cook turkey bacon in a pan until crispy. Remove and set aside.
2. Heat olive oil in the same pan over medium heat.
3. Add the whole eggs and egg whites, scramble gently.
4. Once eggs are nearly set, add spinach and tomatoes and cook briefly until wilted.
5. Chop turkey bacon and fold it into the eggs.
6. Add reduced-fat pepper jack cheese and fold until melted.
7. Season with salt and pepper, to taste.

NUTRITION (Per Serving)

Calories: ~355
Protein: ~38 g
Total Carbohydrates: ~4 g
Dietary Fiber: ~1 g
Sugars: ~2 g
Total Fat: ~20 g
Saturated Fat: ~6 g
Sodium: ~1,000 mg

Breakfast #3 - Avocado Toast with Eggs

This is a simple, reliable breakfast that delivers protein, healthy fats, and sustained energy without overthinking it. It's quick enough for busy mornings but balanced enough to keep you full, focused, and out of the snack drawer for hours. When consistency matters more than creativity, this one always shows up.

Serving Size: 1 serving

INGREDIENTS

- 1 slice bread (Dave's Killer Bread)
- 2 eggs (scrambled or over-easy)
- ½ avocado, sliced

HOW TO MAKE IT:

1. Toast bread.
2. Place bread on a plate.
3. Add eggs onto bread.
4. Spread or layer avocado.
5. Season with sea salt and pepper.

NUTRITION (Per Serving)

Calories: ~370
Protein: ~19 g
Carbohydrates: ~28 g
Fiber: ~8 g
Sugars: ~4 g
Fat: ~22 g
Saturated Fat: ~5 g
Sodium: ~440 mg

Lunch #1 - Adjustable Mixed Greens Salad

The lunch that saved me on busy days, travel days, golf days, and "I don't know what I'm doing in the kitchen" days. This salad is designed to adapt to your day, your appetite, and your training — not the other way around. It works just as well as a light meal, a protein-loaded lunch, or a supporting player next to dinner. When flexibility matters, this one gives you options without sacrificing structure. Eat proudly — this is a clean lunch that keeps you full AND energized.

Serving Size: 4 servings

INGREDIENTS

- 4 ounces spinach
- 4 ounces baby spring mix or baby greens
- 1 medium cucumber, chopped
- 12 cherry tomatoes, halved
- 1 large avocado, sliced
- 1 hard-boiled large egg, chopped
- 2 ounces dried cranberries
- 4 tablespoons mixed nuts
- 2 ounces shredded cheese
- 4 tablespoons raspberry vinaigrette dressing

HOW TO MAKE IT:

1. Fill a large bowl with spinach and mixed greens.
2. Add cucumber and cherry tomatoes.
3. Add avocado and chopped egg.
4. Sprinkle in dried cranberries, mixed nuts, and shredded cheese.
5. Drizzle lightly with raspberry vinaigrette and toss gently.
6. Add your chosen protein based on preference or training needs.

PROTEIN OPTIONS
(Choose One Per Serving)

- Grilled chicken — 3 oz
- Pre-prepared salmon packet — 2.5 oz

NUTRITION STATISTICS — BASE SALAD ONLY
(Per 1 serving — ¼ of total salad, no added protein)

> Calories: ~335
>
> Protein: ~14 g
>
> Total Carbohydrates: ~22 g
>
> Dietary Fiber: ~7 g
>
> Sugars: ~10 g
>
> Total Fat: ~24 g
>
> Saturated Fat: ~6 g
>
> Sodium: ~360 mg

NUTRITION STATISTICS — BASE SALAD

With Grilled Chicken (3 oz)

> Calories: ~475
>
> Protein: ~40 g
>
> Total Fat: ~27 g
>
> Sodium: ~410 mg

With Salmon Packet (2.5 oz / 70 g)

> Calories: ~525
>
> Protein: ~32 g
>
> Total Fat: ~35 g
>
> Sodium: ~610 mg

(Carbohydrates, fiber, and sugars remain consistent with the base.)

Lunch #2 - Healthy Wrap, The Salad's Portable Cousin

This wrap takes the core elements of a solid meal — protein, greens, and flavor — and puts them into a format that works when life is moving fast. It's dependable, customizable, and far better than grabbing whatever's closest when hunger hits.

Serving Size: 1 serving

INGREDIENTS

- Any combination of ingredients from Adjustable Mixed Greens Salad
- Dressing or Dijon mustard (light amount)

HOW TO MAKE IT:

1. Take any or all ingredients from your salad.
2. Add a touch of dressing or Dijon mustard.
3. Place gently into a whole-wheat or low-carb tortilla.
4. Wrap it tightly.
5. Carry discreetly.
6. Eat proudly.

Tortilla: (Add one of the following values to the Base Salad nutrition totals.)

Flour Tortilla (10" standard):
Adds approximately 210 calories, 6 grams of protein, 35 grams of carbohydrates, 2 grams of fiber, 2 grams of sugar, 5 grams of fat, 1.5 grams of saturated fat, and 420 milligrams of sodium.

Whole Wheat Tortilla (10"):
Adds approximately 190 calories, 7 grams of protein, 32 grams of carbohydrates, 4 grams of fiber, 2 grams of sugar, 4 grams of fat, 1 gram of saturated fat, and 380 milligrams of sodium.

Spinach Tortilla (10"):
Adds approximately 180 calories, 6 grams of protein, 30 grams of carbohydrates, 3 grams of fiber, 2 grams of sugar, 4 grams of fat, 1 gram of saturated fat, and 360 milligrams of sodium.

Low-Carb Tortilla:
Adds approximately 70 calories, 5 grams of protein, 18 grams of carbohydrates, 12 grams of fiber, 0 grams of sugar, 3 grams of fat, 1 gram of saturated fat, and 320 milligrams of sodium

Lunch #3 - Mediterranean Salad

Fresh, fast, flavorful — and almost impossible to mess up. This was one of the easiest salads to love. Light, crisp, colorful, and packed with nutrients, this Mediterranean bowl became one of my "I could eat this every day and not get tired of it" lunches. It offers a break from leafy greens while remaining clean, energizing, and deeply satisfying.

Serving Size: 4 servings

INGREDIENTS

- 1 cucumber, striped and chopped
- 1 cup grape tomatoes, halved
- ½ zucchini, peeled and finely chopped
- ⅓ cup sweet onion, finely chopped
- ¼ red bell pepper, finely chopped
- ¼ green bell pepper, finely chopped
- 1 (15 oz) can garbanzo beans, drained
- 1 small can sliced black olives
- 1 tablespoon minced garlic
- ½ teaspoon dried parsley
- ¼ teaspoon dried basil
- ¼ teaspoon sea salt
- 2 tablespoons olive oil
- 2 tablespoons balsamic vinegar
- 2 tablespoons reduced-fat grated Parmesan cheese

PROTEIN OPTIONS
(Choose One Per Serving)

- Grilled chicken — 3 oz
- Turkey breast — 3 oz
- Salmon packet — 2.5 oz
- Feta cheese — 2 oz

HOW TO MAKE IT:

1. Place all vegetables in a large mixing bowl.
2. Add garbanzo beans, olives, garlic, parsley, basil, and sea salt.
3. Drizzle olive oil and balsamic vinegar over the salad and toss gently to combine.
4. Sprinkle it with reduced-fat Parmesan cheese.
5. Add your chosen protein based on preference, season, or training needs.
6. Serve immediately or refrigerate to let flavors develop.

NUTRITION STATISTICS — BASE SALAD ONLY

(Per 1 serving — 4 servings total)

>Calories: ~260
>Protein: ~8 g
>Total Carbohydrates: ~26 g
>Dietary Fiber: ~7 g
>Sugars: ~6.5 g
>Total Fat: ~14 g
>Saturated Fat: ~2.3 g
>Sodium: ~510 mg

NUTRITION STATISTICS — BASE SALAD PLUS

With Grilled Chicken (3 oz)
>Calories: ~400
>Protein: ~34 g
>Total Fat: ~17 g
>Sodium: ~560 mg

With Turkey Breast (3 oz)
>Calories: ~385
>Protein: ~34 g
>Total Fat: ~15.5 g
>Sodium: ~565 mg

With Salmon Packet (2.5 oz)
>Calories: ~450
>Protein: ~28 g
>Total Fat: ~25 g
>Sodium: ~760 mg

With Feta Cheese (2 oz)
>Calories: ~410
>Protein: ~16 g
>Total Fat: ~26 g
>Sodium: ~1,190 mg

Put it in a Pita? A standard pita bread pocket contains approximately 165 calories, 6 grams of protein, 33 grams of carbohydrates, 2 grams of fiber, 1 gram of sugar, 1.5 grams of fat, 0.3 grams of saturated fat, and 320 milligrams of sodium.

SNACKS — SANITY BETWEEN MEALS

Because eating six small meals is easier than pretending you're not hungry. Snacks played a huge role in my success. They kept me fueled without overeating and gave me structure between meals.

Snack #1 - Trader Joe's Chocolate Peanut Butter Protein Bar

This bar became a reliable fallback when real food wasn't an option — especially on long days, travel days, or between meetings. It's sweet enough to feel satisfying but balanced enough to avoid the crash that usually follows sugary snacks. When you need something dependable that won't send your day off the rails, this one earns its place.

Serving Size: 1 bar

How to Make It

1. Open the package on one end.
2. Take a bite.
3. Repeat the process until satisfied.

NUTRITION STATISTICS

Calories: 190
Protein: 10 g
Carbohydrates: 15 g
Fat: 11 g
Fiber: 4 g
Sugars: 8 g
Sodium: 180 mg

Snack #2 - Homemade Protein Balls - Bars

These are my "always ready" bite-sized energy boosters. Perfect for work, the gym, flights, golf, late nights — anywhere you need quick fuel. These are designed for the moments when hunger shows up between meals and discipline gets tested. This snack prevents bad decisions later. My golf buddies always ask if I "brought some extra balls."

Serving Size: 1 Ball or Bar, Full recipe makes 14 Balls or Bars

INGREDIENTS

- 1 cup rolled oats
- ½ cup ground granola
- ½ cup protein powder
- ½ cup dark chocolate chips
- ⅓ cup brown sugar
- ¼ cup flax seed
- 2 tbsp chia seeds
- 2 tbsp hemp seeds
- ¾ cup peanut butter
- ¼ cup honey
- 2 tsp vanilla

HOW TO MAKE IT:

1. Add all dry ingredients to a large bowl and whisk to combine.
2. Add vanilla, honey, and peanut butter.
3. Mix by hand until fully combined. This takes a while — keep going.
4. If texture is an issue, gloves help.

FOR BALLS:

- Roll mixture into evenly sized balls.
- Place on a wax-paper-lined tray.
- Refrigerate for 1 hour to set.

FOR BARS

- Press mixture firmly into a container.
- Cover and refrigerate for 1 hour.
- Cut into portions once set.

Thickness depends on container size.

NUTRITION STATISTICS

Calories: ~260
Protein: ~10 g
Carbohydrates: ~26 g
Fat: ~15 g
Fiber: ~5 g
Sugar: ~15 g
Saturated Fat: ~4 g
Sodium: ~95 m

Snack #3 - Hummus & Cucumber Snack

This is a clean, simple snack that delivers crunch, fiber, and just enough fat to take the edge off hunger. It's light but satisfying, making it perfect for afternoons when you want something fresh instead of packaged. When you need a reset without overeating, this one works.

Serving Size: 1 serving

INGREDIENTS

- 6 tbsp hummus (choose your flavor)
- 1 full cucumber, striped and sliced

HOW TO MAKE IT:

1. Slice the cucumber into rounds or spears.
2. Dip cucumber into hummus.
3. Throw it in your mouth.
4. Repeat until gone.

NUTRITION STATISTICS

Calories: ~180
Protein: ~6 g
Carbohydrates: ~18 g
Fat: ~10 g
Fiber: ~6 g
Sugar: ~5 g
Sodium: ~240 mg

Dinner #1 - Salmon & Veggie Bake

This was one of my earliest go-to dinners because it hit the holy trinity of weeknight meals: Easy to prep — Easy to cook — Easy to clean. This dinner taught me that eating healthy doesn't need to be complicated. Sometimes all you need is a good baking sheet, fresh ingredients, and the willingness to trust the oven.

Serving Size: 1 serving

INGREDIENTS

- 1 farm-raised Atlantic salmon fillet (8 oz, raw)
- ¼ cup broccoli
- ¼ cup asparagus
- ¼ cup cherry tomatoes
- ½ medium Honeycrisp apple, diced
- 2 tablespoons olive oil
- 1 teaspoon salt
- 1 teaspoon black pepper
- Trader Joe's Salmon Rub

HOW TO MAKE IT:

1. Preheat the oven to 400°F.
2. Line a baking sheet with foil or parchment paper.
3. Place salmon on the baking sheet and season with salt, pepper, and Trader Joe's Salmon Rub.
4. Arrange broccoli, asparagus, cherry tomatoes, and diced apple around the salmon.
5. Drizzle olive oil evenly over the salmon and vegetables.
6. Bake for 18–22 minutes, depending on thickness, until salmon is cooked through and flakes easily.
7. Remove from the oven and serve immediately.

NUTRITION STATISTICS

Calories: ~780
Protein: ~47 g
Total Carbohydrates: ~34 g
Dietary Fiber: ~8 g
Sugars: ~18 g
Total Fat: ~52 g
Saturated Fat: ~9 g
Sodium: ~1,550 mg

Dinner #2 - Lemon Pepper Chicken - Instant Pot

This is a clean, protein-first staple designed for maximum flexibility. The lemon pepper keeps the flavor bright and simple, making it easy to pair with rice, quinoa, vegetables, or salads without getting repetitive. It's one of those "cook once, use everywhere" proteins that quietly supports consistency all week long.

Serving Size: 4 servings

INGREDIENTS

- 1 pound raw boneless skinless chicken breast, cut into strips
- 1 tablespoons olive oil
- 1 cup water (for Instant Pot)

Steve's Chicken Rub
(included in nutrition)

- 1 tablespoon lemon pepper
- 1 teaspoon sea salt
- 1 teaspoon garlic powder
- 1 teaspoon onion powder
- 1 teaspoon dried basil
- 1 teaspoon dried oregano
- 1 teaspoon dried parsley
- 1 teaspoon paprika

HOW TO MAKE IT (Instant Pot):

1. Season chicken breast strips generously with Steve's Chicken Rub.
2. Set Instant Pot to Sauté mode and add olive oil.
3. Season chicken breast strips generously with Steve's Chicken Rub.
4. Set Instant Pot to Sauté mode and add olive oil.
5. Lightly sear chicken strips until just golden.

6. Insert the trivet and add water to the bottom of the pot.
7. Place chicken on the trivet.
8. Secure the lid, set the valve to Sealing, and cook on High Pressure for 7-10 minutes.
9. Use a quick release or short natural release.
10. Remove chicken and serve immediately.

NUTRITION STATISTICS

Calories: ~195
Protein: ~31 g
Total Fat: ~7 g
Saturated Fat: ~1.5 g
Total Carbohydrates: ~1 g
Dietary Fiber: 0 g
Sugars: 0 g
Sodium: ~600 mg

OPTIONAL VARIATIONS

Turkey tenderloins instead of chicken. Your favorite lean beef cut. Just don't use my chicken rub on beef. Beef rubs exist for a reason — they're spectacular.

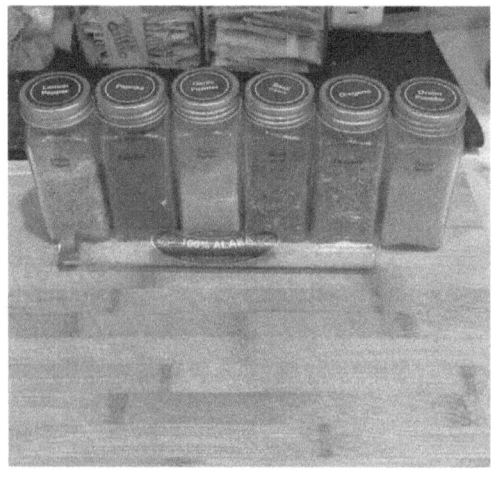

Dinner #3 - Wok Protein & Veggie Bowl

This dinner is so good, it becomes tomorrow's breakfast. Sure, the Instant Pot is John Rambo's Swiss Army knife of the kitchen — powerful, efficient, does 112 things while looking dangerous. But the wok? The wok is Luke Skywalker's lightsaber. It moves fast. It's precise. It sears like a Jedi. And once you learn how to wield it, everything changes. This dinner wasn't just delicious — it taught me how to cook with confidence.

This is the ultimate "build once, eat all week" meal. A big pan of vegetables paired with your protein of choice makes this dish endlessly flexible and easy to adjust based on training demands. It's efficient, satisfying, and one of the most reliable tools in the entire FF50 playbook.

Serving Size: 4 servings

INGREDIENTS - Vegetable Base

- 4-5 broccoli florets
- 4-5 cauliflower florets
- ½ carrot, sliced
- ½ green bell pepper, chopped
- ½ red bell pepper, chopped
- ½ zucchini, chopped
- 4 ounces mushrooms
- 4 ounces spinach
- ½ white onion, diced
- 1 medium jalapeño, finely chopped
- 1 tablespoon minced garlic
- 2 tablespoons olive oil
- 1 teaspoon sea salt
- 1 teaspoon Black Pepper

NUTRITION — BASE ONLY

Calories: ~290

Protein: ~10 g

Total Carbohydrates: ~24 g

Dietary Fiber: ~8 g

Sugars: ~7 g

Total Fat: ~20 g

Saturated Fat: ~3 g

Sodium: ~640 mg

Protein Options
Choose One — 1 pound

- Lean ground turkey (93%)
- Lean ground beef (93%)
- Lean ground chicken
- Shrimp

HOW TO MAKE IT:

1. Heat a wok over medium heat and add olive oil before the pan gets too hot.
2. Add vegetables by density: carrots and broccoli first, then cauliflower, peppers, zucchini, mushrooms, onion, and spinach.
3. Cook, stirring frequently, until vegetables soften and begin to caramelize slightly.
4. Add garlic and jalapeño and cook briefly until fragrant.
5. Season vegetables with salt and pepper.
6. In a separate pan, cook your chosen protein until fully done.
7. Fold cooked protein into the vegetables gently.
8. Serve immediately.

How to Choose Your Protein

This bowl is designed for flexibility, not perfection. Pick your protein based on your day, your hunger level, and your activity.

Leanest option, lowest calories, shrimp is your move.
Maximum protein with moderate fat, chicken or lean ground turkey are your anchors.
Need something more filling, lean ground beef delivers satisfaction without blowing up the system.

Same vegetables, same structure, you choose the fuel that fits the moment.

I prefer to cook the protein in a separate shallow pan — this ensures consistency and allows frozen meat emergencies to be handled gracefully.

NUTRITION STATISTICS — BASE +

With Lean Ground Turkey

    Calories: ~440

    Protein: ~36 g

    Total Fat: ~27 g

    Saturated Fat: ~5 g

    Sodium: ~720 mg

With Lean Ground Beef (93%)

    Calories: ~480

    Protein: ~34 g

    Total Fat: ~32 g

    Saturated Fat: ~9 g

    Sodium: ~730 mg

With Lean Ground Chicken

    Calories: ~410

    Protein: ~39 g

    Total Fat: ~23 g

    Saturated Fat: ~4 g

    Sodium: ~705 mg

With Shrimp

    Calories: ~360

    Protein: ~37 g

    Total Fat: ~21 g

    Saturated Fat: ~3.5 g

    Sodium: ~850 mg

ESTEBAN'S GUAC FOR THE WOK

Some recipes have been shared through whispers in holiday kitchens, passed down for generations, like culinary family folklore. Some recipes are discovered on scattered 3x5 cards in a bread box on grandma's counter. Others hide in an old cookbook dusted with flour and questionable stains, written in cursive so fancy you need a translator to read them.

And then... There are the chosen few revealed on a Chipotle tray liner.

Of all the ancient documents in human history — the Dead Sea Scrolls, the Rosetta Stone — few carry the divine importance of the sacred Chipotle guacamole paper liner. You see, on the day I ordered two tacos, fate delivered me not only lunch... but enlightenment.

Yes, you read that correctly. Printed right there on that liner was Chipotle's official guacamole recipe — playful, confident, and so straightforward that it almost dared me not to try it. So I did. Then I did it again. Then I tweaked a little here, adjusted a little there.

When people started complimenting my guac, I didn't have the heart to tell them it was Chipotle's with a little extra kick.

Serving Size: 2 tablespoons, Makes 8 servings

INGREDIENTS

- 2 large avocados (or 3 medium)
- Juice of ½ lime
- Juice of ½ lemon
- ½ teaspoon sea salt
- Red onion, finely diced
- Fresh cilantro, chopped
- Jalapeño, finely diced
- 2 tablespoons of Organic LOVE

HOW TO MAKE IT:

- Check Avocado ripeness. I read somewhere that they should be about as hard as the thumb muscle inside your palm. I hope that helps you too!

- In a small dish, mix the onion, cilantro, jalapeño, and citrus juice, set aside.
- Slice open Avocados, remove pits.
- Scoop into a mixing bowl.
- Mash with salt.
- Add the "small dish" mixture into the mashed avocado and fold gently.
- Taste.
- Adjust.

NUTRITION STATISTICS

Calories: ~60
Protein: ~1 g
Total Carbohydrates: ~3 g
Dietary Fiber: ~2 g
Sugars: ~0.5 g
Total Fat: ~5 g
Saturated Fat: ~0.8 g
Sodium: ~75 mg

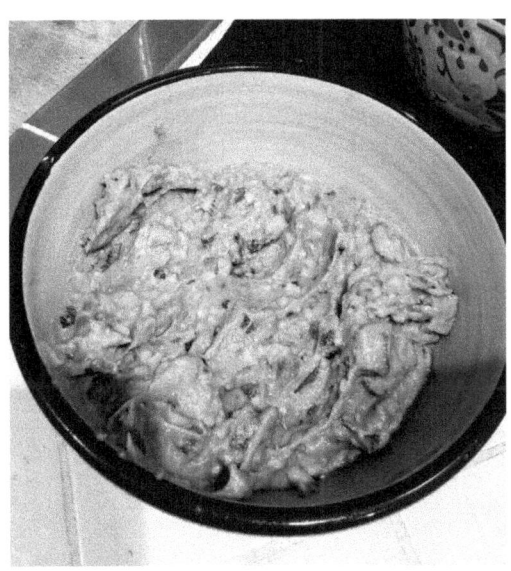

ESTEBAN'S GUAC FOR THE WOK (cont.)

If you're a veteran at eating but new to cooking, let's be honest — tablespoons, ounces, and quarter cups can feel like they're part of a secret kitchen society you forgot to join.

So, here's the good news: **they're all the same here**.

For Esteban's Guac, one serving is:

- ⅛ cup,
- or 1 ounces,
- or 2 tablespoons.

Different words. Same scoop. Same guac.

If you grabbed a measuring cup, great.
If you eyeballed it with confidence, also great.
If you used the same spoon four times and said, "That feels right," congratulations — you're officially cooking.

The goal isn't precision.
The goal is consistency…oh, and not eating the entire bowl straight from the counter.

CHEF'S TIP: Never order avocados online! They will be as hard as baseballs! ASK ME HOW I KNOW!?! Go ahead, ask me!

How to Use It:

On your wok bowl

On a burrito

On toast

On eggs

On your tongue

Straight from the spoon

If anyone tells you that you use too much guacamole, immediately remove them from your life.

No one needs that kind of negativity

THE BONUS BREAKFAST - Leftovers turned legendary.

It is one of the most satisfying, energizing breakfasts I've ever created. This — is how you start your day like a champion.

This breakfast exists to prove that leftovers aren't a compromise — they're a strategy. By folding last night's protein and veggies into a couple of eggs, you get a fast, savory meal that keeps blood sugar steady and cravings quiet. It's efficient, satisfying, and a great reminder that good habits don't have to look like "breakfast food."

Serving Size: 1 serving

INGREDIENTS

- ½ serving of last night's Wok leftovers
- 2 large eggs
- Tbsp olive oil

HOW TO MAKE IT:

1. Heat the wok.
2. Add last night's veggies and protein.
3. Crack in 2 large eggs and scramble them into the mix.
4. Add a spoonful of guacamole on top.

NUTRITION (Per Serving)

Based on ½ serving plus 2 large eggs

Calories: ~480
Protein: ~38 grams
Carbohydrates: ~12 grams
Fiber: ~4 grams
Sugars: ~4 grams
Fat: ~31 grams
Saturated Fat: ~9 grams
Sodium: ~520 milligrams

How to Use This Menu

A simple guide to eating without overthinking it

This chapter is not a diet. It's not a rulebook. And it's definitely not a punishment. It's a menu system. The goal isn't to eat perfectly — it's to eat predictably, consistently, and flexibly, without feeling like food is running your life.

Here's how to use it.

1. Pick a Meal, Not a Math Problem

Every breakfast, lunch, and dinner in this chapter was designed to land in a reasonable calorie range, with solid protein, and enough fat and fiber to keep you full. You don't need to calculate anything day to day.

Pick:

- A protein
- A base
- An optional add-on

Eat. Move on with your life.

2. Repetition Is a Feature, Not a Failure

You'll notice a lot of overlap:

- The same vegetables
- The same proteins
- The same base meals showing up in different forms

That's intentional. Repetition reduces decision fatigue. Decision fatigue is where most people fail. If you eat the same breakfast five days in a row and it works — congratulations, you're doing it right.

3. Swaps Are Safe Inside the System

This menu was built so you can swap without spiraling.

Examples:

- Chicken ↔ turkey ↔ shrimp
- Salad ↔ wrap ↔ bowl
- Avocado ↔ olive oil ↔ guacamole

As long as you stay within the structure, the system holds. You're not "cheating." You're choosing.

4. Portions Matter — But They're Not Fragile

You'll see measurements like:

- 8 oz protein
- ¼ cup guacamole
- 1 tortilla
- ½ serving of leftovers

These aren't traps. They're anchors. You don't need lab-level precision. You need rough consistency over time. If you're close, you're close enough.

5. Bonus Meals Are Built In on Purpose

The Bonus Breakfast exists because:

- Leftovers happen
- Hunger changes
- Real life doesn't follow calendars

Using leftovers + eggs isn't "getting off track." It is the track. The system flexes so you don't break.

6. This Menu Supports Movement — Not the Other Way Around

You don't eat less so you can move. You eat well so movement feels possible. That's why protein stays high. That's why carbs are intentional. That's why fats aren't demonized.

This menu fuels:

- Walking
- Golf
- Stretching
- Long days
- Busy travel
- Low-energy days
- High-activity days

7. If You're Unsure, Default to These Rules

When in doubt:

- Add protein
- Add vegetables
- Keep portions reasonable
- Don't panic
- Eat again later

Consistency beats intensity. Structure beats willpower.

Final Thoughts

This menu isn't here to impress anyone. It's here to make sure that on:

- Busy days
- Travel days
- Low-motivation days
- "I don't feel like thinking" days

You still know exactly what to eat. That's not discipline. That's design. By the time I had mastered these breakfasts, lunches, snacks, and dinners, something unexpected happened. I wasn't just eating better. I wasn't just making better choices. I wasn't just learning recipes. I was building rhythm. I was building momentum. And most importantly…

I was building identity.

Because here's the truth no one tells you. You don't lose weight by force. You lose weight by identity shift. You become someone who cooks at home. Someone who knows exactly what's in their food. Someone who has go-to meals, not just go-to cravings. Someone who can fuel their body without fighting their body.

And for the first time in years, I wasn't just reacting to my hunger or my cravings. I wasn't improvising every day. I wasn't guessing. I had a system. A simple one. A repeatable one. A system that gifted me energy, clarity, flexibility, and a sense of control I had forgotten I could feel.

This chapter wasn't just about meals — it was about the foundation.

The tools. The habits. The mindset. The structure. The identity.

Eating healthy wasn't a punishment at all. It was something I enjoyed. It was something I chose. It was something that made me feel like I was finally aligned with the version of myself I always knew was in there.

And with this foundation in place, I was ready for the next phase.

Every transformation has a moment where you stop warming up and start stepping in. And for me, that moment arrived when I knew I couldn't unsee the fat-face photo. That moment arrived when I knew the habits I built in this chapter were only the preparation. That moment arrived when it was time to do something bold... Something cleansing. Something dramatic. Something that would clear the slate — physically, mentally, emotionally.

It was time for the step that changed everything. It was time to: Get Ready To Get Ready.

The next chapter isn't just about eating better. It's about preparing your body for the 10-Day Master Cleanse, aligning your mindset, and building the 90-day plan that ignited my 50-pound weight-loss transformation.

You've mastered the meals. Now it's time to master the preparation.

CHAPTER FIVE

Get Ready To Get Ready

The Reality Check Nobody Warns You About

If you're going to do the Master Cleanse, there's one thing you need to understand right out of the gate: you are about to go eight and a half days without consuming physical food. Let that land for a second. Eight and a half days. No chewing, no crunching, no nibbling, no "just one bite, it doesn't count." Your jaw is basically going on vacation. And because of this, you can't just wake up on a Tuesday and decide, "Yeah, I think I'll stop eating for a week." This is not a whim cleanse. This is not something you decide spontaneously. This is a calendar event—and if you don't treat it like one, your cleanse will collapse faster than your willpower in the candy aisle at a dollar store.

I know this because the first time I attempted the cleanse with absolutely no planning, it was an epic failure. I thought I could just jump into it, white-knuckle my way through, and come out enlightened on the other side. Nope. By the end of Day Two, I was so hungry I practically sprinted to In-N-Out Burger, bursting through the doors like I had just escaped the wilderness. Cleanse over. Thanks for playing.

That's why the very first rule of cleansing is simple: You cannot do this around major life temptations. Thanksgiving (No way), Christmas (don't even think about it), New Year's Eve (seriously?), your birthday (nope), your significant other's birthday (not unless you want to sleep outside), weddings (a felony cleanse offense), and family vacations (you're kidding, right?). If there is even a remote chance someone will offer you food you love, like, tolerate, or usually avoid but suddenly find irresistible because you haven't eaten in 48 hours—skip that entire week. When you're cleansing, every food becomes sexy.

When I first did the cleanse properly, I thought I understood hunger. I didn't. What I understood was inconvenience—the kind of feeling you get when Starbucks has a long line. Real hunger is different. Real hunger has opinions.

Day 1, I didn't even realize I was cleansing. I was just drinking lemonade like some kind of citrus-obsessed influencer. My only real challenge was getting through the saltwater flush—which we'll discuss in the next chapter, because it deserves its own monologue, a warning label, and possibly a legal disclaimer.

Day 2 is when things got interesting. My stomach figured out we were not playing the usual game. It screamed at me, negotiated with me, and emotionally petitioned for pizza. But every time it yelled "FEED ME," I handed it lemonade instead. And guess what? The hunger went away… briefly. Liquid doesn't stay in your stomach long—it's like, "Thanks for the visit, now get out." So I drank more lemonade and made it through another day.

Then came Day 3. If you've never woken up feeling like a bear coming out of hibernation, congratulations—you've never done this cleanse. I opened my eyes and genuinely considered eating my pillow. Raw. Unseasoned. No regrets. But I stayed strong, did the saltwater flush — and went right back to my lemonade routine.

Somewhere about halfway to two-thirds through Day 3, something changed. The hunger stopped. The pangs went quiet. The voices disappeared. It was like my body finally said, "Oh. This is what we're doing? Okay then. Carry on." The moral of the story? It took three and a half days for my body to get over the psychological connection to physical food. Not the nutritional need—the psychological one. Once my body accepted that I was committed—and that I was, in fact, feeding it in my own strange, lemony way—everything shifted.

And that's why preparation matters. You must set yourself up to survive those first three days, because once you get past the "pillow-eating phase," you're golden.

WHY CLEANSE?

The Surprisingly Logical (and Slightly Embarrassing) Truth About Your Gut**

Most people think digestion is just: food goes in, magic happens, life moves on. But the real story is simpler — and honestly, a little more personal. Your gut is not a passive bystander. Your gut is a training system. Whatever you feed it most often, whatever rhythm you repeat most consistently, that becomes the setting your entire digestive system tunes itself to.

Inside your small and large intestines lives a thin, constantly renewing mucus barrier — a real, biological shield your body builds to protect the single layer of cells standing between your food and your bloodstream. This mucus barrier is supposed to be smooth, balanced, and chill. But when you repeatedly blast your body with greasy fast food, irritating spices, ultra-processed "edible events," and late-night burrito decisions, your gut has to react. And it reacts fast.

When things get sketchy, your body can dump more fluid into your intestines, increase mucus to protect the lining, and speed up everything to flush irritants out. This is why people say, "Taco Bell goes right through me." It's not that Taco Bell hates you. It's that your gut saw something suspicious and hit the button for the internal slip-n- slide.

The real problem is that your gut doesn't say, "Oh hey, broccoli is here — let's slow down and give it the VIP tour." Nope. When your system is trained to operate in high-speed, high-irritation mode, everything rides the same slip-and-slide — even the good stuff. So even when you switch to whole foods, organic lemons, and distilled water like a health monk with decent knife skills, the nutrients don't get the time they deserve. This is where the cleanse comes in.

Let's clear this up: A cleanse does **NOT** peel off ancient rubbery mucoid plaques. What a well-designed cleanse does is calm inflammation, normalize mucus production, reset gut rhythm and transit time, give your microbiome a new script, and allow your body to actually absorb the good stuff you've been eating for three weeks. A cleanse is a reset window, not a punishment. It's your digestive system finally getting to say: "Thank you for stopping the chaos — I can work with this."

By now, you've already cooked real meals, built new habits, practiced consistency, and adopted a healthier identity. The cleanse simply lets your biology sync with your behavior. You've done the work on the outside. This is the moment you support the shift on the inside.

Mental, Emotional, and Logistical Readiness

Before you begin the Master Cleanse, you have to understand that this isn't just a physical process. It's not just "stop eating and see what happens." If that were the case, everyone who ever got stuck in an airport for seven hours would come out looking like a fitness model. No—this cleanse requires three layers of readiness: mental, emotional, and logistical. Miss any one of these, and you're setting yourself up for a rematch with In-N-Out Burger.

Mental Readiness: Deciding You're Actually Doing This

Mental readiness begins with a decision—not a maybe, not a "let's see how it goes," not a soft launch like you're testing out a new Instagram filter. You must make a clear internal agreement with yourself: *I am doing the cleanse.* Because your brain is going to test that agreement the moment you get hungry, bored, emotional, tired, annoyed, nostalgic, lonely, happy, or within smelling distance of a bakery. Mental readiness is integrity. If you don't anchor the decision now, you'll negotiate it later—and trust me, hunger is a world-class negotiator. You need a clean, final, no-turning-back commitment. Once the decision is locked, everything else becomes easier... not easy, but easier.

Emotional Readiness: Understanding the Food-Mood Connection

Next comes emotional readiness, which is where most people underestimate themselves. We tend to forget that food is emotional. It's comfort, reward, distraction, celebration, sedation, therapy, entertainment, tradition, habit, and sometimes an Olympic sport. When you stop eating for eight and a half days, you're not just removing calories—you're removing your coping system.

On Day 2, when your stomach starts sounding like a wounded dinosaur, your emotions will want to panic. On Day 3, when you wake up ready to eat the decorative soaps in your guest bathroom, your emotions will want to revolt. Emotional readiness means knowing this will happen…and choosing to stay with the process anyway. You're not suppressing emotions—you're simply refusing to let them drive the car while they're in a full meltdown.

Emotional readiness is the moment you understand: *I will feel things. This is normal. This is expected. This is temporary. And most importantly: This is not an emergency.*

Logistical Readiness: Setting Up Your World So You Can Win

Finally, we have logistical readiness, which is the grown-up side of the cleanse. This is where you prepare your environment, your schedule, and your daily life so you're not fighting unnecessary battles. Because here's the truth: if you start the cleanse in the middle of a stressful work week, an overloaded schedule, or a family event where someone always shows up with warm cookies, you are not setting yourself up to succeed. You are setting yourself up to fail spectacularly—and probably with crumbs on your face.

Logistical readiness means clearing your calendar of temptations, planning your shopping trips, setting aside time for daily prep, making sure you're not traveling, and ensuring you're sleeping in your own bed. It means not starting a cleanse the same week your boss announces a "mandatory team bonding happy hour," or when your cousin decides to host a taco night. It means being honest about what's happening in your life and choosing a window where nothing is actively trying to sabotage you.

When your mental commitment is solid, your emotional expectations are realistic, and your logistical environment is set, the cleanse becomes far less overwhelming. These three layers work together to get you through the hardest part—the beginning—so that your body can shift into the rhythm it needs for the rest of the journey.

What You Already Built in Chapter 3

Before you begin any cleanse, especially one as intense as the Master Cleanse, it's important to recognize what you've already accomplished. Chapter 3 wasn't just a collection of recipes and menu plans—it was your training camp. It was your warm-up lap. It was the part where you learned how to nourish yourself with intention instead of improvisation. And that matters, because the body you bring into the cleanse is the body that will carry you through it.

Most people fail cleanses because they jump into them straight from chaos. They go from "I haven't cooked a real meal in six months" to "Let me just stop eating entirely," and then wonder why their body riots on Day 2. But you? You already did the work. You went through the three-week cooking trial period. You learned how to prepare fresh meals. You built consistency. You created predictable fuel instead of last-minute food emergencies. All of that has stabilized your body and your mind.

When you spent three weeks making your breakfasts, lunches, snacks, and dinners, you were doing far more than following recipes—you were building an identity. You became someone who plans, someone who cooks, someone who knows exactly what's in their food and why it's there. That identity shift is powerful. It teaches your body and brain that you are capable of caring for yourself, that you can be trusted with your own wellbeing. And this trust becomes the foundation for the cleanse.

Your new cooking skills also serve another purpose: they create a metabolic landing strip. Instead of jumping from fast food and takeout into a zero-calorie liquid diet, you've adjusted your body to cleaner ingredients, lower inflammation, and more stable energy. This makes the entry into the cleanse smoother. It reduces the shock. It shortens the chaos window of Days 1–3. You've already begun the detox without realizing it.

Even more importantly, by practicing the meal plan from Chapter 3, you've already demonstrated your ability to follow a system. Cleansing isn't about willpower—it's about rhythm. Routine. Execution. You've shown yourself that you can follow steps, maintain structure, and trust the process. The Master Cleanse is simply the next progression of that system.

So as you prepare to transition into the cleanse, take a moment to acknowledge that you're not starting from scratch. You've laid the groundwork. You've built habits. You've created momentum. And you are far more prepared for this journey than you might think.

Choosing the Right Cleanse Window

Choosing your cleanse window is one of the most important—and most overlooked—parts of the entire Master Cleanse experience. Most people treat scheduling like an afterthought, as if the cleanse is something you can wedge between errands, meetings, and emotional landmines. But this is not a dental appointment. This is not "swing by and pick up dry cleaning." This is eight and a half days without food, which means timing is everything.

When you choose your cleanse window, think of yourself as a pilot choosing a runway. You can't just land anywhere. You need space, clarity, good weather, and preferably no emotional turbulence. Because here's the truth: the cleanse doesn't care about your calendar—but your calendar will absolutely sabotage your cleanse if you're not intentional.

First, eliminate the obvious no-fly zones. The big holidays—Thanksgiving, Christmas, New Year's Eve—are out. Birthdays are out too: yours, your family's, your partner's, your coworker's, that neighbor you barely know but somehow always ends up serving cake. Weddings are out. Vacations are out. Any event with a buffet? Immediate disqualification.

But it's not just the major temptations you need to avoid. Stress matters. Energy matters. Emotional load matters. If you're in a high-pressure period at work, dealing with personal upheaval, hosting guests, or navigating anything that already strains your bandwidth, this is not the time to also stop eating for over a week. You want a window where your life feels stable—boring, even. A cleanse thrives in boring conditions. Boring is your friend.

At the same time, don't overthink your calendar to the point where it becomes impossible to find a window at all. This isn't a military operation. Maintaining your lemonade diet is not the most difficult thing in the world—it's simply something you want to set up as thoughtfully as possible. The goal is not perfection; the goal is to choose a reasonable, supportive stretch of days where you can focus on yourself without unnecessary distraction or temptation. Life will never hand you a flawless week, but it will absolutely hand you a workable one.

The ideal cleanse window is a ten-day stretch (eight and a half days of cleansing plus your exit days) where you have minimal social obligations, no travel, no parties, no big decisions, and no major temptations. You're not hiding from life—you're simply clearing space for a temporary, purposeful reset. You're carving out a clean lane for your mind and body to do exactly what they need to do without being ambushed by cake, work stress, or taco night.

And here's the part people rarely consider: your mindset matters just as much as your schedule. If you go into the cleanse feeling overwhelmed, burnt out, or emotionally stretched thin, those first three days will feel like you're swimming upstream with ankle weights on. But if you enter with preparation, focus, and a clear window, your chances of success skyrocket.

Choosing the right cleanse window is an act of self-leadership. It's you saying, *"I'm giving myself the conditions to win."* And once you do, everything that follows—the prep, the shopping, the daily routine—becomes dramatically more manageable.

Why Timing Matters

Timing is one of the most underestimated elements of the Master Cleanse. People think success comes down to willpower, discipline, grit, or how long they can stare at a sandwich without crying. But the truth is, timing has a far bigger impact on your cleanse than your willpower ever will. If you begin the cleanse during the wrong week, the wrong emotional season, or the wrong life moment, your body and brain will put up resistance that feels ten times harder than it needs to be.

When your stress is high, your cravings are high. When your schedule is overloaded, your patience is low. When your energy is scattered, your hunger feels louder. Starting a cleanse under those conditions is like attempting to meditate in the middle of a construction site. Can it be done? Technically, yes. Should you try it? Absolutely not.

That's why timing matters. You're giving your body space to transition gently instead of yanking the rug out from under it at the worst possible moment. If you start on a week where your emotions are already stretched, every hunger pang feels like a crisis. If you start on a week where you're overwhelmed at work, every lemonade feels like a chore. And if you start during a social week filled with dinners, birthdays, cocktails, and "You've gotta try this," then you're not cleansing—you're tempting fate.

Timing also matters because your body follows rhythms. Energy, digestion, sleep cycles, hormones, mental clarity—they all move in patterns. When you choose a calm window, those rhythms support you instead of fight you. The cleanse becomes an aligned experience rather than an uphill battle.

But here's the bigger, deeper truth: choosing the right timing tells your brain that this cleanse is important. It communicates seriousness. It communicates intention. When you carve out a dedicated window, you're signaling to yourself, *I'm prioritizing my health. I'm not squeezing this in—I'm making space for it.* That internal alignment makes a massive difference in how you experience the first few days, which are always the toughest.

Think of the cleanse like launching a rocket. The launchpad has to be stable or the whole mission fails. You don't want outside forces shaking you off the pad before you even get going. A calm window gives your mind, your body, and yes, your stomach, the smoothest possible runway for takeoff.

In other words: timing isn't everything… but it's close.

Shopping Lists, Planning & Expectation-Setting

Once you've chosen your cleanse window, the next step is gathering your supplies. Now, for some people, grocery shopping is a normal human activity. For others, it's a stressful expedition into a fluorescent-lit maze where hope goes to die. If you fall into the second category, don't worry—I've designed this preparation process to keep your excitement high and your overwhelm low.

First, let's talk about the big three items that are easier—and frankly, more fun—to order online: your cayenne tablets, your Dark, Thick & Robust maple syrup, and your Smooth Move evening tea. I personally order these from Amazon before the cleanse begins. It's not just convenient; it builds momentum. There's something about seeing those packages show up at your door that makes you feel like, *Yes. I am actually doing this.* It turns preparation into anticipation, like you're gearing up for a mission rather than dreading a chore.

Once those items are on the way, your first trip to the store becomes extremely simple. All you need to grab are distilled water, organic lemons, and sea salt (if you don't already have it). That's it. Three things. And let me be incredibly clear here: it **must** be distilled water. Not spring water. Not filtered water. Not tap water. Not Aquafina. Not Evian—yes, I know it spells "naïve" backwards, and yes, that's clever, but still no. Distilled water only. This cleanse is about giving your body a break, not giving it a chemistry experiment in every glass.

And while we're clarifying non-negotiables: your lemons must be organic. Non-organic lemons come with pesticides, wax coatings, mystery chemicals, and whatever else they decided to spray on them that week. You do not want that in your system when you're trying to detox. Organic lemons only. Period. Don't cleanse your body with pesticide lemonade—we're trying to get healthier, not accidentally pickle ourselves from the inside.

Now, here's a key strategy: do not buy all your organic lemons at once. Yes, you're going to need a lot of them. Yes, you're going to be squeezing lemons like it's your part-time job. But even the best organic lemons get bruised, soften, or start looking like they've questioned their life choices after four or five days. Freshness matters. So only buy enough lemons for the first half of the cleanse. Your second lemon run will happen around Day 4—conveniently timed right after you've survived the Day 3 sanity challenge and suddenly feel like a superhero.

That second trip is where the excitement really kicks in. Because on Day 4, wandering into the grocery store is a completely different experience. You've made it through the hardest part. You're mentally sharp, physically lighter, and emotionally proud of yourself. That trip feels like an achievement. You'll buy your second batch of organic lemons, and you'll also pick up everything you need for your exit days—specifically your orange juice (not from concentrate) and all the fresh vegetables for your Day 9 vegetable soup.

No recipe spoilers yet, but trust me: that soup will taste like gourmet heaven after what you just accomplished.

This two-phase shopping strategy—Amazon delivery, simple first store run, celebratory second store run—not only makes logistical sense, it also keeps your enthusiasm alive. You're breaking the prep into manageable steps. You're reducing stress. You're building anticipation. And the whole experience becomes something you're engaged with, rather than something you're surviving.

Expectation-setting is also crucial here. The first few days of the cleanse will be an adjustment—your hunger will speak up, your emotions might get dramatic, and your brain will do its best to convince you that chewing is a human right. But once you get past that early turbulence, the process becomes clear, steady, and surprisingly energizing. Preparing your supplies in advance ensures that during those tougher moments, you are not scrambling. You're not debating whether to run to the store. You're simply following the system and staying on track.

With your supplies ready, your expectations aligned, and your environment set up to support you, you're now prepared for the final step: getting your body and mind ready for the cleanse itself.

Preparing Your Body and Mind for the Master Cleanse

The days leading up to the cleanse are just as important as the cleanse itself. This is the part most people skip, which is why most people fail. They think the cleanse starts on Day 1, but the truth is that the cleanse starts before Day 1. How you treat your body and mind in the days leading up to the cleanse determines whether those first three days feel like a manageable adjustment... or like you've been dropped into a survival show with no training and no snacks.

You Already Did the Hardest Part

Before we go any further, take a moment to acknowledge something important: you've already spent three weeks building your new kitchen practice. You learned how to cook for yourself. You created structure. You consistently fueled your body with real ingredients and intentional meals. This is the foundation every cleanse hopes for—but almost no one actually has.

And here's the beautiful truth: you don't have to be perfect. Maybe you improvised. Maybe you had a few slip-ups. Maybe you burned something (or everything). That doesn't matter. What matters is that you progressed. You built rhythm. You built awareness. You built a relationship with your own food choices. Now is the moment when all of that preparation comes together. The cleanse is not a cold restart—it's the next chapter in a process you've already begun. Your body is primed. Your mindset is aligned. Your habits have momentum. You're not entering the cleanse from chaos; you're entering from stability.

Hydration: Don't Start the Cleanse Dehydrated

Hydration before the cleanse is crucial. If you show up to Day 1 already dehydrated, your body is going to send you complaint notes. So in the days leading up, drink plenty of water—this doesn't mean gallons, but enough that your body isn't running on fumes. The saltwater flush will be easier, your energy will be steadier, and your brain won't feel like it's being powered by a cracked iPhone battery.

Sleep: Don't Begin the Cleanse Exhausted

There is a massive difference between cleansing while well-rested and cleansing while exhausted. Starting the cleanse tired is like starting a marathon with one shoe missing. Get your sleep in order before you begin. Go to bed a little earlier. Reduce stimulating late-night activities. Give your body the restoration it needs so it can focus on detoxing rather than just trying to keep you upright.

Light Movement: Wake Up Your Circulation

You don't need to train for a triathlon. You don't need to suddenly become a yogi. But you do want some light movement in the days leading up to the cleanse. A few short walks. Some stretching. Maybe a gentle workout if that's your thing. You're not trying to burn calories—you're trying to get your circulation moving so your body isn't shocked when the detox begins.

Reduce Your Mental Load

Part of preparing your body is preparing your brain. The fewer decisions you have to make during the first few days of the cleanse, the better. Finish lingering tasks. Clear off your desk. Handle small responsibilities now so they don't show up on Day 2 when your stomach is already auditioning for a horror movie soundtrack. A calmer mind equals a smoother cleanse.

Set Your Agreements With Yourself

One of the most powerful parts of preparation is establishing personal agreements—simple rules you commit to following no matter what. Things like:

-When I'm hungry, I drink.
When I panic, I breathe.
When I crave something, I remind myself it's temporary.
When I doubt myself, I remember why I started.

These agreements are your anchor during the days when emotion and hunger try to negotiate against your goals.

Reset Your Environment: Remove Temptation and... Leftovers

This step is essential: clean your kitchen before the cleanse begins. Remove snacks, comfort foods, unfinished desserts, and anything that whispers your name at 11 p.m. And here's the big one—make sure all leftovers have either been eaten or donated to someone who is not you. Because when you're cleansing and your brain starts looking for excuses, "I shouldn't waste food" suddenly becomes a full moral argument.

You'll convince yourself that eating the leftover pasta is a heroic act of reducing waste, that finishing the last slice of pizza is basically saving the planet. No. That is the cleanse brain trying to trick you. Do not leave temptation in the refrigerator. Eat the leftovers, give them to the dog, drop them at a neighbor's house—whatever you need to do, make sure they are gone.

Earn Your Body's Trust

This preparation phase is more than logistics—it's about building trust with your body. When you hydrate properly, rest well, move lightly, clarify your commitments, and clean your environment, you're sending a message: *You're safe. I've got you. We're doing this together.* That trust will carry you through the hardest days of the cleanse and help your body shift into cooperation instead of resistance.

Once your body and mind feel supported, the cleanse stops being a battle and becomes a process—a challenging one, yes, but a doable, purposeful, and transformative one. Preparation is the bridge between intention and execution, and now you're ready to step onto that bridge.

Preparation Leads To Action

By this point, you've done something most people never do: you've actually prepared. Not pretend prepared. Not "I watched a YouTube video and feel spiritually ready" prepared. You have done the real work. You built kitchen skills. You stabilized your meals. You created rhythm, awareness, and consistency over three weeks. Then you layered on the mental, emotional, and logistical pieces. You cleared your calendar. You ordered your supplies. You prepped your environment. You even eliminated the leftover spaghetti so it wouldn't seduce you on Day 2.

This chapter wasn't just about getting ready—it was about becoming someone who takes ownership of their own process. Someone who doesn't wing it. Someone who doesn't just hope for success but actually sets up the conditions for it. Someone who recognizes that a cleanse isn't punishment, and it isn't magic—it's a practice of intention, structure, and self-respect.

And now, because of the work you've done, you're stepping into the Master Cleanse with momentum instead of fear. Confidence instead of chaos. You're not going in blind—you're going in equipped, informed, and ready for the journey.

Chapter 5 is where we take all of this preparation and put it into real action. We'll walk through the cleanse itself day by day, including exactly how to make your lemonade, how to handle the hunger waves, and yes, the full breakdown of the saltwater flush—which deserves both an instruction manual and a support group.

You're ready. You've built your foundation. It's time to move from preparation… to transformation.

CHAPTER SIX

The Seven-Day Master Cleanse

The reset cleanse that rebooted everything.

Sometimes in life, you don't need a new workout plan, a fancy supplement, or a celebrity-endorsed hack. Sometimes you need a reset— a clean slate, a full-system reboot, a hard "control-alt-delete" for your digestive, emotional, and decision-making systems. That's what the Master Cleanse became for me.

But before we go any further, let me say this: This cleanse is simple. This cleanse is powerful. This cleanse is… controversial. Some people swear it changed their life. Some swear it ruined a weekend. Some think it's a cult with lemons. For me? It was the turning point. The Clean Break. The Reset.

What the Master Cleanse Actually Is
(Minus the Internet Panic)

At its core, the Master Cleanse consists of four key pieces:

- Morning saltwater flush
- Homemade lemonade mixture throughout the day
- Cayenne Pepper capsules
- Nightly herbal laxative tea.

That's it. No food. No chewing. No exceptions. You're giving your digestive system a break—like sending it on a 10-day spa retreat, except the spa is inside your abdomen and plays ocean sounds at very inappropriate volumes.

But the cleanse isn't about starvation. It's about resting the system, breaking old cravings, resetting your relationship with food, cleaning out years of buildup, building discipline, and creating momentum. I didn't start it looking for enlightenment. I started it because my body needed a reset and because I was ready—finally ready—to become someone different.

Why It Works (Digestive Reset + Visceral Fat Logic)

Before we talk about how the cleanse feels, let's talk about why it works. You've heard me talk about mucus buildup in the intestines. Over decades, your body lines the inside of your digestive tract with little protective pockets—mucoid patches—that act like a slip-and-slide. This makes bad food rush through ("Taco Bell goes right through me!"), but unfortunately, it also reduces absorption of the good stuff.

So the cleanse does three things: gives digestion a break, gently disrupts and dissolves old buildup, and resets your cravings and absorption capacity.

Carpenter's Insight: The Reverse Sandpaper Analogy

Picture a carpenter working with raw wood. Before they can turn it into a masterpiece, they sand it down: heavy grit, medium grit, fine grit. Only then is the surface ready for paint, stain, or sealant. Now imagine your intestines... but in reverse.

The Master Cleanse uses mild internal "abrasives" like cayenne pepper, citric acid from lemons, and the saltwater flush—not to scrape, but to loosen, soften, and gently remove the old residue. You're not sanding the wood to shape it—you're removing old finishes so the new finish can actually bond. That's what this cleanse does: It prepares your digestive system for the amazing food you're about to feed it.

The Master Cleanse Menu & Daily Routine (Your Exact Protocol)

Here is the exact daily routine I followed—simple, strict, and effective.

Morning — The Salt Water Flush

- 2 pints distilled water (find the temperature that works for you)
- 1 teaspoon sea salt in each pint
- Chug both (I plug my nose)
- Stay near a bathroom (see story below)

Pro Tip: Right after you chug the saltwater, you get about 20 minutes before the internal fireworks begin. This window is PERFECT for preparing your full gallon of lemonade for the day. The productivity is satisfying… and it gives the bathroom sprint more emotional dignity.

Daily Lemonade (Drink Whenever Hungry)

- 1 gallon distilled water
- 1 cup organic lemon juice
- 1 cup dark, thick, robust maple syrup
- Cayenne tablets: 1 tablet, 3–4x daily

Now, let's talk about doing the cleanse when you actually have things to do outside your home. Because unless you've scheduled a personal 10-day monastery retreat, you're going to need a plan.

Key things you need

- Your favorite sports bottle, something easy to drink from.
- A large plastic pitcher for your refrigerator.
- Two or three large mason jars with tight-sealing lids
- A soft-shell travel cooler with freezable ice packs.

When you make your lemonade, pour the full batch into your pitcher and let any overflow go into the mason jars. When you leave the house, fill your sports bottle. If you know you'll be gone longer—like a full day of work—pour extra lemonade into the mason jars, seal them, pack them in your cooler, and take them with you.

The key is making sure you have enough lemonade for however long you'll be out, because once you leave your home… you leave your kitchen. And you're not going to find this lemonade at Whole Foods, Amazon Fresh, or even Trader Joe's. This lemonade must be made by you, packed by you, and traveled with you.

Evening

- 1 cup Smooth Move organic tea
- Stevia optional
- Do not skip this

Wheatgrass: The Optional Sidekick

Whether you're a fan or you think it tastes like something a cow chewed, reconsidered, and returned for store credit, I strongly recommend a two-ounce wheatgrass shot each morning. It calms hunger, boosts nutrients, supports detox, and fits within cleanse guidelines. It's optional, but it's powerful. And yes, Jamba Juice was my dealer.

Medical Note

Get standard bloodwork before starting the cleanse. Then go again a couple months after. The improvement might shock you.

My First Saltwater Flush Story

On Day 1 of my first cleanse, I started with the *Salt Water Flush*. After choking down 32 ounces of salt water. I sat down to play a little online poker while waiting for the saltwater to "do its thing." About twenty minutes later, I felt a little bubble—a familiar sensation, the kind confidently handled by a man with 40-plus years of farting experience. So I released what I believed would be a gentle squeaker.

It was not. It was… squishier.

My bathroom is 11 paces away. I know this because each pace was accompanied by another sound—like my body was signaling Morse code for "You fool." As I started to sit down, a pressurized stream of liquid blasted out of me with the enthusiasm of a burst hydrant. Not diarrhea. No. Diarrhea is gentle compared to this.

The sensation was so bizarre I started laughing, which only intensified the sprinkler-effect rhythm echoing off the bowl. And this is how I learned the golden rule of the Master Cleanse:

Golden Rule: Never Trust a Fart!

Accountability & Partnership (Why You Didn't Quit)

I don't recommend attempting the Master Cleanse alone. People start it alone. But finishing? That takes a partner. Daily check-ins. Daily "Are you alive?" texts. Daily "Don't you dare quit on me" talks. On Day 3, we both wanted to quit—but neither of us wanted to be the first to admit it. That mutual stubbornness was the glue that held us together.

Accountability builds identity. Identity builds consistency. Consistency builds transformation.

The Emotional & Physical Timeline (Days 1-10)

Your real experience, not the Internet version.

Day 1 — Cute, Fun, and Completely Misunderstood

Day 1 is adorable. You think the cleanse is an adventure. The lemonade tastes good. You're excited. You have no idea what's coming. The saltwater flush humbles you, but still—you think, "I got this." Day 1 is a lie. But you don't know that yet.

Day 2 — Reality Arrives

Now you know what the saltwater tastes like, what the flush feels like, and what a fart really is (a threat). Your brain starts objecting: "You should be eating today. Humans eat daily." Day 1 felt like an anomaly. Day 2 proves it wasn't. At some point, you WILL think: "Where's the beef?"

Day 3 — The Hardest Day

Day 3 hits like a freight train. I woke up wanting to eat my pillow. My stomach was folding itself like origami. And I learned another lesson the hard way: Drink lemonade before bed. If you don't, you WILL pay the price. But somewhere in the middle of Day 3, everything changes. The psychological addiction to food breaks. Your mind quiets down. Your body adapts. You cross the threshold most people never reach.

Day 4 — Motivation, Momentum, and Overconfidence

On Day 4, I felt superhuman. I suggested extending the cleanse to 10 days and then turning it into a 2-week detox. My partner said, "I agreed to 7 days. I'm doing 7 days." Seven days turned out to be perfect. But Day 4 teaches you something powerful: Your brain starts trusting you again. You begin seeing possibilities you couldn't see before. Identity shift is happening.

Day 5 — Calm, Clarity, Beauty Everywhere

Day 5 is peace. You feel lighter, brighter, energized. Flowers smell different. Food commercials no longer own your soul. You feel in control of yourself for the first time in a long time.

Day 7 — A Cathartic Final Push

When Day 7 arrives, it feels like the end of an emotional marathon. You're proud, centered, stronger than your cravings. Every hunger pang, every emotional dip, and every moment you peed out of your butt… worth it.

Day 8 — The Exit Begins (50/50 OJ + Soup Prep Magic)

Day 8 is the start of the exit: 50% orange juice and 50% water or lemonade. You feel transformed. Your stomach is calm. Your identity is different. The evening of Day 8 is when you prepare your vegetable soup. You return to the kitchen like a warrior entering a temple. Your chopping skills come back immediately. The vegetables look brighter, fuller, almost glowing. And this is one time—and ONE TIME ONLY—that I tell you not to use the Instant Pot. Use the crock pot. Slow cook. Eight hours. Overnight. Trust me.

Day 9 — The Best Morning Smell of Your Life

When you wake up on Day 9, the entire house is filled with the aroma of your soup. You haven't even gotten out of bed yet, and it feels like breaking through a finish-line ribbon. The smell is emotional. The taste is spiritual. Your self-trust is at an all-time high.

Day 10 — Reintroduction Without Cravings

On Day 10, you reintroduce real food. But here's the transformation: You don't crave sugar. You don't crave carbs. You don't crave the foods that used to own you. Your digestive system is clean. Your brain is recalibrated. Your cravings belong to YOU again. The factory reset is complete.

Resetting Cravings (The Digestive "Factory Reset")

The cleanse doesn't just detox your body—it reboots your taste buds. Suddenly sugar is too sweet, processed foods taste fake, and natural foods taste incredible. Your body begins telling the truth again. And you can finally hear it.

Exiting the Cleanse (Critical)

Day 1 of Exit (Day 8 total)

50/50 orange juice + distilled water or lemonade.

Day 2 of Exit (Day 9 total)

50/50 orange juice + vegetable soup.

Day 3 of Exit (Day 10 total)

Begin your new menu plan.

This is where people make the biggest mistakes. Exiting the cleanse is NOT where you celebrate with pizza. You must land the plane gently. This step dramatically helps determine your long term results.

The Unexpected Wins

By the end of the cleanse, you notice your mind is quieter, your cravings are calmer, your confidence is higher, your discipline is stronger, and your identity has shifted. This isn't a diet. It's a declaration—a declaration that you are ready to reset, release old habits, and become someone powerful, someone who honors their body, someone who trusts themselves, someone who's ready for what comes next.

Day Nine - The Organic Vegetable Soup (Crock Pot)

WELCOME BACK FOOD! This soup isn't about nutrition perfection or protein targets. It's about **re-entry**. After the 50/50 OJ day, your body doesn't need to be challenged — it needs to be welcomed back. Organic

Vegetable Soup (Crock Pot) is the soft landing. You start it before bed, let it cook while you sleep, and wake up to a house that smells like calm, warmth, and the quiet confidence of someone who made a good decision yesterday.

I debated whether to include serving sizes or nutrition information for this recipe — and for this recipe only. The reason is simple. This day isn't about tracking numbers. It's about celebrating completion. It's about honoring the journey and the value of what you just gave your body. If you choose to start counting numbers and worrying about macros again today, I support that completely. But in my opinion, today follows just two rules: **eat when you're hungry, and eat until you're full.** No spreadsheets. No math. Just trust. This is how you tell your system, *we're good — and we're moving forward.*

For today only, there are no macros to hit and nothing to track. Eat when you're hungry. Stop when you're full. You've earned that

The Organic Vegetable Soup

Serving Size: HUNGER

INGREDIENTS

- 8 cups low-sodium vegetable broth
- 1 (28 oz) can crushed tomatoes
- 8 oz garbanzo beans, drained
- ½ cup green beans
- ½ red pepper, chopped
- ½ green pepper, chopped
- ½ large onion, chopped
- 1 medium potato, diced
- 1 green apple, chopped
- 1 pear, chopped
- 1 rib celery, diced
- 1 large carrot, diced
- ½ small zucchini, diced
- 3 cloves garlic, minced
- 1 tbsp fresh parsley, minced
- 1 tbsp dried oregano
- 1 tsp dried thyme
- ½ tsp fresh ground black pepper

HOW TO MAKE IT:

1. Combine all ingredients in a slow cooker.
2. Gently stir everything together.
3. Cook on low for 8 hours.

NUTRITION - Per 8-Ounce Serving

Calories: ~65 kcal
Protein: ~2.5 g
Carbohydrates: ~14.5 g
Fiber: ~3.5-4 g
Total Fat: ~0.5 g
Saturated Fat: ~0.1 g
Sugar (naturally occurring): ~7 g
Sodium: ~110 mg

Crock Pot Size Note

This recipe fits comfortably in an 8-quart slow cooker.
In a 6-quart slow cooker, it will fit very full at the start and should not exceed the manufacturer's maximum fill line. The vegetables will cook down significantly within the first hour.

Yield & Serving Information

- Total cooked volume: ~140 oz
- Serving size: 8 oz
- Number of servings: ~17–18

CHAPTER SEVEN

90-Day Gameplan

Meals, Movement, and Momentum

This is the moment where structure creates transformation.

There's a moment in every health journey when you ask yourself, "Okay… now what?" Not dramatically. Not an existential crisis. More like the moment after successfully building Ikea furniture and thinking, "Look at that—I did it. It only wobbles when you touch it." This is exactly what the 90-Day Game Plan answers.

This chapter isn't about suffering, self-denial, or becoming the person who suddenly starts jogging at sunrise. It's about something far more effective: structure. Structure creates rhythm. Rhythm creates consistency. Consistency creates momentum. Momentum creates transformation.

And the entire system rests on three pillars: Meals. Movement. Momentum. Master these, and you don't just change—you become someone new.

SECTION ONE: MEALS

How to eat like someone who knows what they're doing.

You've already built a foundation with Chapter 3. You have your breakfasts, lunches, and dinners that don't require a panic attack or twelve minutes of staring into the fridge like it holds the secrets of the universe. But the next 90 days aren't about what you can cook. They're about removing decisions.

Because nothing derails healthy eating faster than standing in the kitchen at 6:07 p.m. wondering if mustard qualifies as dinner.

This section builds the meal system that eliminates that moment.

ADDING NEW IDEAS TO CHAPTER 3'S RECIPES

You're not rebuilding your diet from scratch. You're expanding it—purposefully and intelligently. You already have your foundation. Now we take things to the next level.

During my own five-month transformation, I kept a detailed log of every single meal I ate. Not because I thought I'd be writing a book someday, but because I wanted to know what actually worked—and why. What kept me consistent. What kept me satisfied. What kept me moving toward my goals without burning out.

And here's the exciting part: I'm going to give you that entire menu. Every breakfast. Every lunch. Every dinner. Every go-to meal. Every fallback meal. Every "this saved me when life got crazy" recipe.

You can follow my menu exactly, pick and choose your favorites, mix, match, rotate, customize based on your tastes and schedule, or ignore anything that doesn't work for you. Your job isn't to become a gourmet chef. Your job is to create a system—a weekly rotation of meals you love, that you'll actually eat, that doesn't require daily decision-making.

Because the meals you eat consistently… consistently move you toward your goals.

And here's your teaser: In the next chapter, I will lay out the full five-month menu exactly as I ate it. Everything laid out, ready for you to use or adapt. Consider this your preview. The full menu is on its way.

- WEEKLY MEAL TEMPLATES

Meal templates eliminate negotiation and stress.

Universal Weekly Template:
- Breakfast: Two rotating favorites
- Lunch: A simple three-day cycle
- Dinner: Protein + vegetable + one weekly variation meal

My Real Template:
- Breakfast: Eggs + avocado or smoothie
- Lunch: Chicken bowl → Mediterranean salad → leftovers
- Dinner: Steak night, chicken night, salmon night, pasta replacement night

Templates bring peace. Peace creates consistency.

- GROCERY RHYTHMS

Grocery shopping isn't a quest. It's a loop. Pick meals → Buy the same ingredients → Restock before emergencies. Predictable groceries make eating well automatic.

- REMOVING DECISION FATIGUE

People don't fail diets. People fail daily decision-making under stress. Your 90-day structure erases that.

SECTION TWO: MOVEMENT

Move like someone who wants their joints working at 70.

Movement doesn't need to be complicated. It doesn't require a gym, a trainer, a cult-like 5 a.m. class, or a subscription to workouts designed for Olympians. It requires three things: Walking. Stretching. Consistency.

Simple wins.

- WALKING: THE MOST UNDERRATED EXERCISE

Walking improves everything. It burns calories, reduces stress, boosts mood, improves digestion, clears your mind, and anchors identity. If all you did for 90 days was walk, your body would change dramatically.

- STEP GOALS: 10K → 12K → 14K

Build gradually:

- Month 1: 10,000
- Month 2: 12,000
- Month 3: 14,000

Your metabolism stands at attention at 14k.

- GOLF AS MOVEMENT, NOT LEISURE

Golf counts—if you walk it. And how you walk it matters more than you think.

For years, I used a push cart. I thought that made me look organized, athletic, maybe even pro-level-adjacent. Then a chiropractor told me, "Pushing a golf cart is the worst way to walk the course."

He explained, "When you push a cart, you're locking your elbows." "You're locking your shoulders."

"You're leaning forward."
"You're putting tension in your lower back."
"You're shoving a weighted object in front of your body in ways humans weren't designed to move."

Basically, I was recreating the posture of someone trying to push a stalled pickup truck uphill.

Then he told me, "The second worst way to golf is in a golf cart."

Not only do you skip all the steps, but most golf cart suspensions are ornamental. You bounce around like two cans of paint in a Home Depot shaking machine. Your kidneys deserve better.

So what's the best way? "Walk with a carry bag."

A walking bag distributes weight evenly, mimics a backpack, supports natural posture, preserves your gait, and turns golf into a scenic walk with occasional bursts of athletic frustration.

After switching from a push cart to a carry bag, I loved golf more. My back felt better. My steps increased. The game became a movement practice instead of a slow-motion kidney assault.

Obviously, if you have back or foot issues, adjustments should be made. This isn't dogma—it's optimization. But if you can walk and carry, your body will thank you.

- ## P90X STRETCH / YOGA-FLOW STRETCHING

Here's the secret most people overlook: mobility accelerates weight loss. Tight muscles slow you down. Inflamed joints slow you down. Restricted movement slows you down. Stretching fixes all of that. But let me tell you how my stretching journey began.

The first time I did P90X Stretch, I watched the people on screen bend like warm taffy. They weren't just touching their toes—they were palms down behind their feet, sometimes using yoga blocks to stretch even farther. Meanwhile, I was struggling to barely touch my toes. I genuinely believed flexibility was genetic.

Wrong again.

With consistent stretching—daily or even every other day—things changed fast. The combination of stretching, the cleanse, and an anti-inflammatory diet opened up my joints, lengthened my muscles, and made walking easier. Because flexibility isn't just muscle. It's hinges—hips, shoulders, knees.

Reduce inflammation → hinges open.
Hinges open → muscles lengthen.
Muscles lengthen → movement increases.
Movement increases → transformation accelerates.

And at some point you'll say, "Why didn't I start stretching years ago?"

- HOW MOVEMENT ANCHORS IDENTITY

Movement doesn't just shape your body. It shapes who you believe you are. Walk and you become a walker. Stretch and you become flexible. Golf for steps and you become someone who chooses movement.

Identity is always greater than discipline.

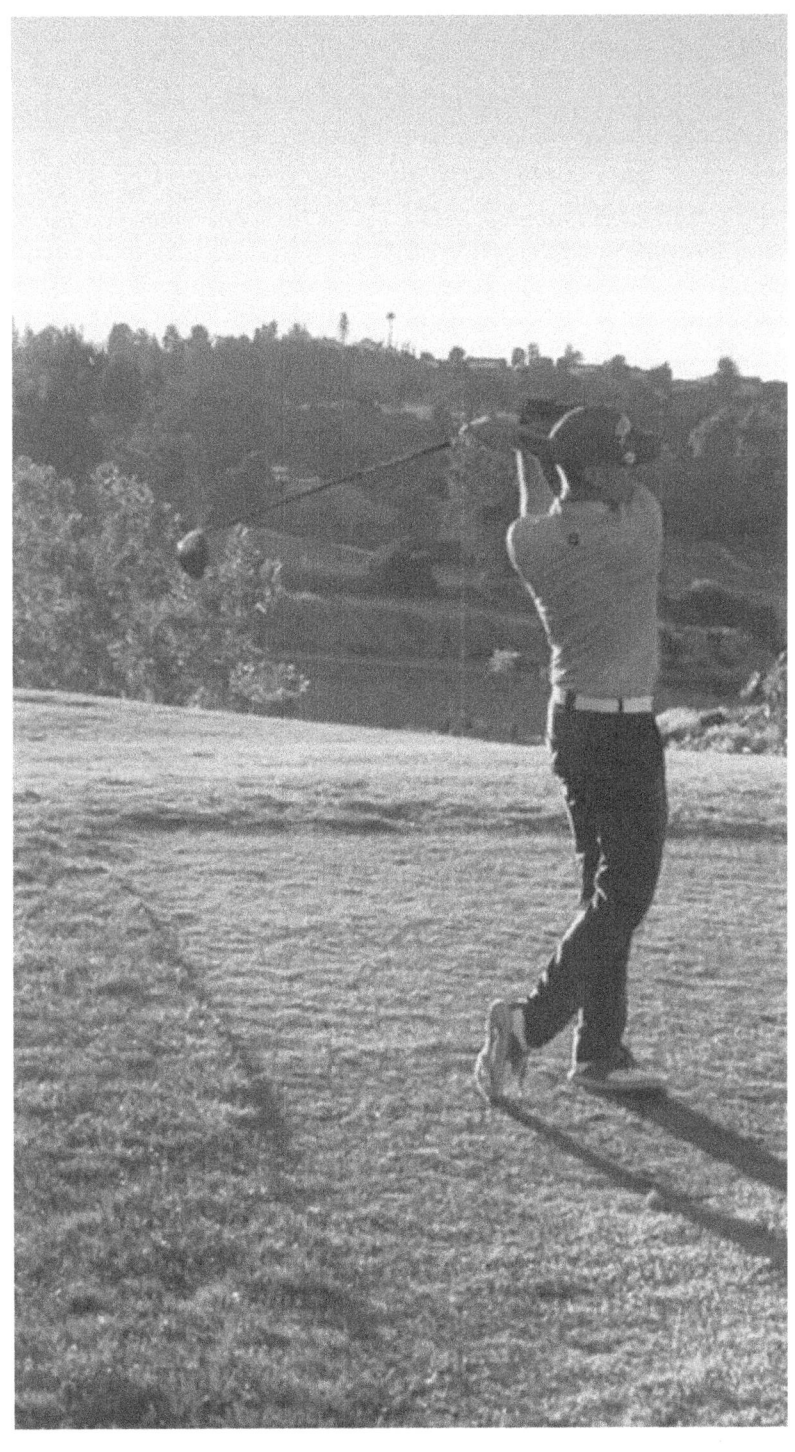

SECTION THREE: MOMENTUM

The psychology of staying in motion. Momentum isn't magic. Momentum is physics and psychology working together. You've heard the saying, "An object in motion stays in motion. An object at rest stays at rest." People think that's physics. And it is. But it's also your Tuesday.

Momentum is what happens when you maintain just enough movement that stopping feels unnatural. The next 90 days train you to stay in motion.

- DAILY CONSISTENCY MINDSET

Forget perfect days. You need present days. Your new rule: "Just do something." Something keeps you in motion. Nothing stops everything.

- ACCOUNTABILITY STRUCTURES

Accountability isn't punishment. It's support.

Use anything that helps you stay honest:
- Friends
- Calendars
- Step trackers
- Journals
- Coaches
- Weekly check-ins

Anchors prevent drift.

- TRACKING WITHOUT OBSESSION

Tracking builds awareness, not guilt. Track steps, sleep, water, meal patterns, weekly trends.

I personally used MyFitnessPal. Not because it's magic. Not because it's perfect. And not because I want to become a MyFitnessPal coach. I used it because it made the math easy.

Apps like this let you set clear goals for calories, protein, carbohydrates, and fats. They show you numbers instead of guesses. They remove mental math from your brain.

But the real value isn't just tracking what's coming in. It's also tracking what's going out.

Most apps allow you to log your activity. When I would go out early in the morning and walk nine holes of golf, I would log that movement. The app would then increase my available calorie intake for the day.

That's when everything really clicked.

It wasn't just about eating less. It was about balancing one side of the equation with the other. Calories in versus calories out. Movement versus fuel.

That math was what allowed me to truly dial in weight loss while still making sure I was getting enough protein, enough carbohydrates, and enough good fats to support my body.

On days when you work out hard, you get to enjoy more food. The math reflects the effort. You move more, your body needs more, and the system supports that instead of fighting it.

And on days where work or the schedule gets the best of you and you aren't able to be as active, there's relief in knowing that your intake still matched your needs for that day. No punishment. No guilt. Just alignment.

You stop wondering.
You stop guessing.

You stop adjusting emotionally.
You adjust logically.

The key here is restraint. You don't need to track forever. You don't need to track every bite. You don't need perfection. You just need awareness long enough to understand your patterns.

Think of it like using a GPS. You don't stare at it every second, but it's helpful to know you're still headed in the right direction.

Use whatever app you like. Use it temporarily or seasonally. Use it until things click. Then put it down.

The goal isn't tracking.
The goal is alignment.

- THE PSYCHOLOGY OF "JUST DO SOMETHING"

Your brain rewards completion. Do something small, and your brain proudly declares, "We're someone who follows through." That identity fuels more action.

- MOTIVATION AS THE RESULT OF ACTION

Motivation doesn't begin the transformation. Action does.

Action → motivation → more action.

That loop is the engine of your momentum.

- ACTING LIKE THE PERSON YOU WANT TO BECOME

For the next 90 days, you behave like someone who moves, someone who eats intentionally, someone who tracks without shame, someone who doesn't negotiate with excuses, and someone who finishes.

This isn't pretending. This is a rehearsal.

Rehearsal becomes identity. Identity becomes your new normal.

The 90-Day Game Plan isn't a diet. It isn't a challenge. It's the architecture of transformation.

Meals. Movement. Momentum.
Simple. Sustainable. Repeatable.

Follow the system and it carries you. Stay in motion and momentum meets you. Act like the person you want to become... and eventually, inevitably, you are them.

CHAPTER EIGHT

The Fit and Flexible Recipe Library

The meals that did the heavy lifting.

Meals are like thoughts. The good ones can lift you up, give you energy, and make you feel empowered. The bad ones have the potential to quickly take your day off the rails.

Breakfast gets skipped or rushed. Lunch is reactive. Snacks are whatever is closest. And by the time dinner rolls around, you are tired, hungry, and negotiating with yourself like it is a hostage situation. "I'll just have a little." "I earned this." "Tomorrow I'll be better."

This chapter exists to end that pattern.

Before you ever get here, you've already done important work. Those first weeks weren't about restriction — they were about learning. You practiced cooking. You got comfortable in your kitchen. You figured out what you actually like to eat. Not what you're supposed to like. What you like.

A lot of recipes say things like salt and pepper, to taste. That phrase used to annoy me. To taste? Whose taste? And then something clicked: to taste means you have to taste it. You cook it. You try it. You adjust it. And suddenly, you know. That's not a throwaway instruction — that's the skill.

That moment matters more than people think. Because once you've tasted, adjusted, and enjoyed your own food, you stop needing someone else to tell you what works. You start trusting yourself.

With those skills in place, this chapter opens up. Breakfast becomes something you can rely on. Lunch becomes adjustable instead of chaotic. Snacks stop feeling like mistakes. And dinner — the meal that used to break people — becomes manageable, repeatable, and even enjoyable.

Everything in this chapter is built from meals I've cooked, eaten, tweaked, and shared — sometimes alone, sometimes with friends, sometimes with family sitting around the table. These aren't theoretical recipes. They're real meals that had to work in real life.

Use these meals as written, or treat them like frameworks. Swap flavors. Adjust portions. Add protein when you need it. Skip what doesn't work. The goal isn't perfection — it's consistency.

Because when food stops being a daily negotiation and starts becoming something you understand, the rest of the process gets easier.

Chapter 8 — Recipe Library

Breakfast

Avocado Toast and Eggs	101
The Protein Shake	102
TJ's Acai Bowl	104
Turkey Bacon, Eggs and Spinach Scramble	105
The Bonus Breakfast — Wok Leftovers + Eggs	106

Lunch

Adjustable Mixed Greens Salad	108
Healthy Wrap	110
Mediterranean Salad	111
Street Tacos	113
TJ Falafel Salad	114

Snacks

Homemade Protein Balls	116
Hummus & Cucumber Snack	117
Trader Joe's Chocolate Peanut Butter Protein Bar	118

Dinner

Baked Southwest Chicken	120
Chicken Primavera Spaghetti Squash Boats	121
Chicken Vegetable Casserole	123
Creamy Spinach Spaghetti Squash Casserole	125
Honey Garlic Chicken (Instant Pot)	127
Lemon Pepper Chicken (Instant Pot)	128
Mexican Cauliflower Rice Casserole	130
Mexican Chicken and Cauliflower Rice Casserole	132
Orange Chicken - Air Fryer	133
Pork Carnitas (Instant Pot)	135
Pot Roast and Potatoes (Instant Pot)	137

Salmon & Veggie Bake	139
Sesame Chicken and Veggies — Sheet Pan	140
Shrimp Scampi	142
Spaghetti Squash with Meat / Vodka Sauce	143
Spinach Stuffed Chicken Breasts	147
Stuffed Eggplant with Chicken	149
Thai Chicken Coconut Curry	151
Thai Red Curry with Vegetables	153
Thai Red Curry with Chicken	155
Tilapia and Veggies	156
(Healthy) Tuna Noodle Casserole	157
Wok Protein & Veggie Bowl	159

Other / Sides

Esteban's Guacamole	161

BREAKFAST

Avocado Toast with Eggs

This is a simple, reliable breakfast that delivers protein, healthy fats, and sustained energy without overthinking it. It's quick enough for busy mornings but balanced enough to keep you full, focused, and out of the snack drawer for hours. When consistency matters more than creativity, this one always shows up.

Serving Size: 1 serving

INGREDIENTS

- 1 slice bread (Dave's Killer Bread)
- 2 eggs (scrambled or over-easy)
- ½ avocado, sliced

HOW TO MAKE IT:

1. Toast bread.
2. Place bread on a plate.
3. Add eggs onto bread.
4. Spread or layer avocado.
5. Season with sea salt and pepper

NUTRITION (Per Serving)

Calories: ~370
Protein: ~19 g
Carbohydrates: ~28 g
Fiber: ~8 g
Sugars: ~4 g
Fat: ~22 g
Saturated Fat: ~5 g
Sodium: ~440 mg

Breakfast #1 - Super Fruit Protein Shake

This is the quick morning shake that jump-started my transformation. It is the ultimate no-excuses breakfast for mornings when time is tight but standards are still high. It's built to deliver solid protein, fiber, and nutrients in one smooth move, without leaving you hungry an hour later. Think of it as a reliable bridge between "I should eat" and "I have five minutes."

Serving Size: 1 serving

INGREDIENTS

- 8-10 oz unsweetened vanilla almond milk
- 1½ scoops protein powder
- ½ frozen banana
- 1 tablespoon peanut butter
- ¼-⅓ cup frozen mixed berries (raspberry/blackberry/blueberry combo)
- ¼ cup frozen spinach
- 1 tablespoon chia seeds
- 1 teaspoon creatine

NUTRITION (Per Serving)

Calories: ~448
Protein: ~44 g
Carbohydrates: ~34 g
Fiber: ~9 g
Sugars: ~13 g
Fat: ~17 g
Saturated Fat: ~4-5 g
Sodium: ~470 mg

HOW TO MAKE IT:

7. Add almond milk to the Magic Bullet.
8. Toss in frozen banana.
9. Add peanut butter.
10. Add protein powder, creatine, and chia seeds.
11. Add berries.
12. Blend until smooth.

Refreshing Fruit Variation

It's built to deliver solid protein, fiber, and nutrients in one smooth move, without leaving you hungry an hour later. The pineapple–mango version keeps things light and refreshing.

INGREDIENTS

- Swap berries for: Frozen pineapple, frozen mango, or both

NUTRITION (Per Serving)

>Calories: ~452
>Protein: ~44 g
>Carbohydrates: ~36 g
>Fiber: ~6 g
>Sugars: ~19 g
>Fat: ~17 g
>Saturated Fat: ~4–5 g
>Sodium: ~470 mg

Chocolate Peanut Butter Option

The chocolate peanut butter option tastes like a Chocolate Peanut Butter cup that somehow still supports your goals.

INGREDIENTS

- 8–10 oz almond milk
- 1½ scoops chocolate protein powder
- ½ frozen banana
- 1 tablespoon peanut butter
- 1 teaspoon creatine

NUTRITION (Per Serving)

Calories: ~428
Protein: ~44 g Fiber: ~4 g
Sugars: ~12 g
Fat: ~15 g
Saturated Fat: ~4 g
Sodium: ~320 mg

TJ's Acai Bowl

This is the breakfast that feels indulgent but still plays by the rules. It's cold, refreshing, and satisfying, with enough protein and fiber to keep it from turning into a sugar crash. When you want something that feels like a treat but still supports your goals, this bowl earns its spot.

Serving Size: 1 serving

INGREDIENTS

- ½ packet Trader Joe's Acai Puree Packet
- ½ scoop vanilla whey protein powder
- 1 medium banana
- ½ cup mixed berries (blackberry, raspberry, blueberry)
- 1 tablespoon creamy peanut butter
- 1 teaspoon ground flaxseed
- 1 teaspoon chia seeds
- ¾ cup (170 g) Chobani Plain Non-Fat Greek Yogurt
- 2 tablespoons unsweetened vanilla almond milk
- 3 tablespoons Trader Joe's granola
- 1 tablespoon organic honey

HOW TO MAKE IT:

1. Add the acai puree and banana to a blender.
2. Add protein powder, mixed berries, peanut butter, flaxseed, chia seeds, Greek yogurt, and almond milk.
3. Blend until thick and smooth.
4. Pour into a bowl.
5. Top with granola.
6. Drizzle with honey and serve immediately.

NUTRITION STATISTICS

Calories: ~485
Protein: ~26 g
Total Carbohydrates: ~63 g
Dietary Fiber: ~19 g
Sugars: ~33 g
Total Fat: ~17 g
Saturated Fat: ~3.5 g
Sodium: ~170 mg

Turkey Bacon, Eggs & Spinach Scramble

This is a high-protein, low-nonsense breakfast that hits hard without feeling heavy. It's fast, filling, and flexible — perfect for mornings when you want real food, real energy, and zero decision fatigue. If you're training, traveling, or just trying to stay on track, this scramble does the job.

Serving Size: 1 serving

INGREDIENTS

- 6 slices turkey bacon
- 2 large whole eggs
- 4 additional large egg whites
- ⅓ cup spinach
- 4 cherry tomatoes, halved
- ¼ cup reduced-fat pepper jack cheese
- 1 teaspoon olive oil
- Salt, to taste
- Pepper, to taste

HOW TO MAKE IT:

1. Cook turkey bacon in a pan until crispy. Remove and set aside.
2. Heat olive oil in the same pan over medium heat.
3. Add the whole eggs and egg whites, scramble gently.
4. Once eggs are nearly set, add spinach and tomatoes and cook briefly until wilted.
5. Chop turkey bacon and fold it into the eggs.
6. Add reduced-fat pepper jack cheese and fold until melted.
7. Season with salt and pepper, to taste.

NUTRITION (Per Serving)

Calories: ~355
Protein: ~38 g
Total Carbohydrates: ~4 g
Dietary Fiber: ~1 g
Sugars: ~2 g
Total Fat: ~20 g
Saturated Fat: ~6 g
Sodium: ~1,000 mg

Wok Leftovers + Eggs — Bonus Breakfast

It is one of the most satisfying, energizing breakfasts I've ever created. This — is how you start your day like a champion.

This breakfast exists to prove that leftovers aren't a compromise — they're a strategy. By folding last night's protein and veggies into a couple of eggs, you get a fast, savory meal that keeps blood sugar steady and cravings quiet. It's efficient, satisfying, and a great reminder that good habits don't have to look like "breakfast food."

Serving Size: 1 serving

INGREDIENTS

- ½ serving of last night's Wok leftovers
- 2 large eggs
- Tbsp olive oil

HOW TO MAKE IT:

5. Heat the wok.
6. Add last night's veggies and protein.
7. Crack in 2 large eggs and scramble them into the mix.
8. Add a spoonful of guacamole on top.

NUTRITION (Per Serving)

Based on ½ serving plus 2 large eggs

Calories: ~480
Protein: ~38 grams
Carbohydrates: ~12 grams
Fiber: ~4 grams
Sugars: ~4 grams
Fat: ~31 grams
Saturated Fat: ~9 grams
Sodium: ~520 milligrams

LUNCHES

Adjustable Mixed Greens Salad

The lunch that saved me on busy days, travel days, golf days, and "I don't know what I'm doing in the kitchen" days. This salad is designed to adapt to your day, your appetite, and your training — not the other way around. It works just as well as a light meal, a protein-loaded lunch, or a supporting player next to dinner. When flexibility matters, this one gives you options without sacrificing structure. Eat proudly — this is a clean lunch that keeps you full AND energized.

Serving Size: 4 servings

INGREDIENTS

- 4 ounces spinach
- 4 ounces baby spring mix or baby greens
- 1 medium cucumber, chopped
- 12 cherry tomatoes, halved
- 1 large avocado, sliced
- 1 hard-boiled large egg, chopped
- 2 ounces dried cranberries
- 4 tablespoons mixed nuts
- 2 ounces shredded cheese
- 4 tablespoons raspberry vinaigrette dressing

HOW TO MAKE IT:

1. Fill a large bowl with spinach and mixed greens.
2. Add cucumber and cherry tomatoes.
3. Add avocado and chopped egg.
4. Sprinkle in dried cranberries, mixed nuts, and shredded cheese.
5. Drizzle lightly with raspberry vinaigrette and toss gently.
6. Add your chosen protein based on preference or training needs.

PROTEIN OPTIONS
(Choose One Per Serving)

- Grilled chicken — 3 oz
- Pre-prepared salmon packet — 2.5 oz

NUTRITION STATISTICS — BASE SALAD ONLY
(Per 1 serving — ¼ of total salad, no added protein)

    Calories: ~335

    Protein: ~14 g

    Total Carbohydrates: ~22 g

    Dietary Fiber: ~7 g

    Sugars: ~10 g

    Total Fat: ~24 g

    Saturated Fat: ~6 g

    Sodium: ~360 mg

NUTRITION STATISTICS — BASE SALAD

    With Grilled Chicken (3 oz)

    Calories: ~475

    Protein: ~40 g

    Total Fat: ~27 g

    Sodium: ~410 mg

With Salmon Packet (2.5 oz / 70 g)

    Calories: ~525

    Protein: ~32 g

    Total Fat: ~35 g

    Sodium: ~610 mg

(Carbohydrates, fiber, and sugars remain consistent with the base.)

Healthy Wrap, The Salad's Portable Cousin

This wrap takes the core elements of a solid meal — protein, greens, and flavor — and puts them into a format that works when life is moving fast. It's dependable, customizable, and far better than grabbing whatever's closest when hunger hits.

Serving Size: 1 serving

INGREDIENTS

- Any combination of ingredients from Adjustable Mixed Greens Salad
- Dressing or Dijon mustard (light amount)

HOW TO MAKE IT:

1. Take any or all ingredients from your salad.
2. Add a touch of dressing or Dijon mustard.
3. Place gently into a whole-wheat or low-carb tortilla.
4. Wrap it tightly.
5. Carry discreetly.
6. Eat proudly.

Tortilla: (Add one of the following values to the Base Salad nutrition totals.)

Flour Tortilla (10" standard):
Adds approximately 210 calories, 6 grams of protein, 35 grams of carbohydrates, 2 grams of fiber, 2 grams of sugar, 5 grams of fat, 1.5 grams of saturated fat, and 420 milligrams of sodium.

Whole Wheat Tortilla (10"):
Adds approximately 190 calories, 7 grams of protein, 32 grams of carbohydrates, 4 grams of fiber, 2 grams of sugar, 4 grams of fat, 1 gram of saturated fat, and 380 milligrams of sodium.

Spinach Tortilla (10"):
Adds approximately 180 calories, 6 grams of protein, 30 grams of carbohydrates, 3 grams of fiber, 2 grams of sugar, 4 grams of fat, 1 gram of saturated fat, and 360 milligrams of sodium.

Low-Carb Tortilla:
Adds approximately 70 calories, 5 grams of protein, 18 grams of carbohydrates, 12 grams of fiber, 0 grams of sugar, 3 grams of fat, 1 gram of saturated fat, and 320 milligrams of sodium

Mediterranean Salad

Fresh, fast, flavorful — and almost impossible to mess up. This was one of the easiest salads to love. Light, crisp, colorful, and packed with nutrients, this Mediterranean bowl became one of my "I could eat this every day and not get tired of it" lunches. It offers a break from leafy greens while remaining clean, energizing, and deeply satisfying.

Serving Size: 4 servings

INGREDIENTS

- 1 cucumber, striped and chopped
- 1 cup grape tomatoes, halved
- ½ zucchini, peeled and finely chopped
- ⅓ cup sweet onion, finely chopped
- ¼ red bell pepper, finely chopped
- ¼ green bell pepper, finely chopped
- 1 (15 oz) can garbanzo beans, drained
- 1 small can sliced black olives
- 1 tablespoon minced garlic
- ½ teaspoon dried parsley
- ¼ teaspoon dried basil
- ¼ teaspoon sea salt
- 2 tablespoons olive oil
- 2 tablespoons balsamic vinegar
- 2 tablespoons reduced-fat grated Parmesan cheese

PROTEIN OPTIONS
(Choose One Per Serving)

- Grilled chicken — 3 oz
- Turkey breast — 3 oz
- Salmon packet — 2.5 oz
- Feta cheese — 2 oz

HOW TO MAKE IT:

1. Place all vegetables in a large mixing bowl.
2. Add garbanzo beans, olives, garlic, parsley, basil, and sea salt.
3. Drizzle olive oil and balsamic vinegar over the salad and toss gently to combine.
4. Sprinkle it with reduced-fat Parmesan cheese.
5. Add your chosen protein based on preference, season, or training needs.
6. Serve immediately or refrigerate to let flavors develop.

NUTRITION STATISTICS — BASE SALAD ONLY

(Per 1 serving — 4 servings total)

    Calories: ~260
    Protein: ~8 g
    Total Carbohydrates: ~26 g
    Dietary Fiber: ~7 g
    Sugars: ~6.5 g
    Total Fat: ~14 g
    Saturated Fat: ~2.3 g
    Sodium: ~510 mg

NUTRITION STATISTICS — BASE SALAD PLUS

With Grilled Chicken (3 oz)
    Calories: ~400
    Protein: ~34 g
    Total Fat: ~17 g
    Sodium: ~560 mg

With Turkey Breast (3 oz)
    Calories: ~385
    Protein: ~34 g
    Total Fat: ~15.5 g
    Sodium: ~565 mg

With Salmon Packet (2.5 oz)
    Calories: ~450
    Protein: ~28 g
    Total Fat: ~25 g
    Sodium: ~760 mg

With Feta Cheese (2 oz)
    Calories: ~410
    Protein: ~16 g
    Total Fat: ~26 g
    Sodium: ~1,190 mg

Put it in a Pita? A standard pita bread pocket contains approximately 165 calories, 6 grams of protein, 33 grams of carbohydrates, 2 grams of fiber, 1 gram of sugar, 1.5 grams of fat, 0.3 grams of saturated fat, and 320 milligrams of sodium.

Street Tacos

These tacos are proof that simple, familiar food can still fit inside a smart routine. Lean protein, just enough fat, and controlled portions make this a satisfying meal without turning into a calorie spiral. It's a great reminder that balance doesn't mean giving things up — it means building them correctly.

Serving Size: 3 Tacos

INGREDIENTS

- 3 Mission white corn street taco tortillas
- 4 oz ground turkey
- 1 tbsp olive oil
- 2 tbsp picante sauce
- 1 oz shredded Mexican cheese
- 2 tbsp fresh cilantro, chopped
- ¼ cup white onion, finely chopped

HOW TO MAKE IT:

1. Heat olive oil in a pan over medium heat.
2. Add ground turkey and cook until fully browned.
3. Stir in the chopped white onion and cook for 1-2 minutes until softened.
4. Warm tortillas in a dry pan.
5. Spoon cooked turkey mixture evenly into each tortilla.
6. Top with shredded cheese.
7. Add picante sauce.
8. Sprinkle with chopped cilantro.
9. Fold and serve.

NUTRITION (Per Serving)

Calories: ~505
Protein: ~34 g
Carbohydrates: ~26 g
Fat: ~33 g
Fiber: ~4 g
Sugar: ~4 g
Sodium: ~560 mg

TJ Falafel Salad

This salad brings bold flavor and crunch without tipping into "junk food disguised as healthy." It's hearty enough to stand on its own, but still clean and controlled when portions matter. When you want something satisfying and different that doesn't derail your day, this one delivers.

Serving Size: 1 serving

INGREDIENTS

- 0.42 cup Trader Joe's Falafel Mix, baked
- 2 cups romaine lettuce
- 1 Persian cucumber, sliced
- 1 tablespoon crispy jalapeños
- 2 tablespoons light ranch dressing

HOW TO MAKE IT:

1. Prepare the falafel mix according to package directions and bake.
2. Chop the romaine lettuce and add to a bowl.
3. Slice the Persian cucumber and add to the salad.
4. Add baked falafel on top.
5. Sprinkle with crispy jalapeños.
6. Drizzle with light ranch dressing.
7. Toss lightly or eat layered.

NUTRITION (Per Serving)

Calories: ~505
Protein: ~34 g
Carbohydrates: ~26 g
Fat: ~33 g
Fiber: ~4 g
Sugar: ~4 g
Sodium: ~560 mg

SNACKS

Homemade Protein Balls - Bars

These are my "always ready" bite-sized energy boosters. Perfect for work, the gym, flights, golf, late nights — anywhere you need quick fuel. These are designed for the moments when hunger shows up between meals and discipline gets tested. This snack prevents bad decisions later. My golf buddies always ask if I "brought some extra balls."

Serving Size: 1 Ball or Bar, Full recipe makes 14 Balls or Bars

INGREDIENTS

- 1 cup rolled oats
- ½ cup ground granola
- ½ cup protein powder
- ½ cup dark chocolate chips
- ⅓ cup brown sugar
- ¼ cup flax seed
- 2 tbsp chia seeds
- 2 tbsp hemp seeds
- ¾ cup peanut butter
- ¼ cup honey
- 2 tsp vanilla

HOW TO MAKE IT:

1. Add all dry ingredients to a large bowl and whisk to combine.
2. Add vanilla, honey, and peanut butter.
3. Mix by hand until fully combined. This takes a while — keep going.
4. If texture is an issue, gloves help.

FOR BALLS:

- Roll mixture into evenly sized balls.
- Place on a wax-paper-lined tray.
- Refrigerate for 1 hour to set.

FOR BARS

- Press mixture firmly into a container.
- Cover and refrigerate for 1 hour.
- Cut into portions once set.

Thickness depends on container size.

NUTRITION STATISTICS

Calories: ~260
Protein: ~10 g
Carbohydrates: ~26 g
Fat: ~15 g
Fiber: ~5 g
Sugar: ~15 g
Saturated Fat: ~4 g
Sodium: ~95 mg

Hummus & Cucumber Snack

This is a clean, simple snack that delivers crunch, fiber, and just enough fat to take the edge off hunger. It's light but satisfying, making it perfect for afternoons when you want something fresh instead of packaged. When you need a reset without overeating, this one works.

Serving Size: 1 serving

INGREDIENTS

- 6 tbsp hummus (choose your flavor)
- 1 full cucumber, striped and sliced

HOW TO MAKE IT:

1. Slice the cucumber into rounds or spears.
2. Dip cucumber into hummus.
3. Throw it in your mouth.
4. Repeat until gone.

NUTRITION STATISTICS

Calories: ~180
Protein: ~6 g
Carbohydrates: ~18 g
Fat: ~10 g
Fiber: ~6 g
Sugar: ~5 g
Sodium: ~240 mg

Trader Joe's Chocolate Peanut Butter Protein Bar

This bar became a reliable fallback when real food wasn't an option — especially on long days, travel days, or between meetings. It's sweet enough to feel satisfying but balanced enough to avoid the crash that usually follows sugary snacks. When you need something dependable that won't send your day off the rails, this one earns its place.

Serving Size: 1 bar

HOW TO MAKE IT:

1. Open the package on one end.
2. Take a bite.
3. Repeat the process until satisfied.

NUTRITION STATISTICS

Calories: 190
Protein: 10 g
Carbohydrates: 15 g
Fat: 11 g
Fiber: 4 g
Sugars: 8 g
Sodium: 180 mg

DINNERS

Baked Southwest Chicken

When you want something hearty, balanced, and easy to portion for leftovers, this is a simple, flavor-packed dinner that comes together with minimal effort and big payoff. It's loaded with protein, colorful vegetables, and just enough cheese to feel satisfied.

Serving Size: 4 servings

INGREDIENTS

- 1 pound boneless skinless chicken breast
- 1 can black beans, rinsed and drained
- 1 cup corn
- 2 bell peppers, chopped
- 1 cup cherry tomatoes
- ¼ onion, chopped
- 1 portobello mushroom
- 1 jalapeño
- Juice of ½ lime
- 1 cup Colby Jack cheese, shredded
- ½ teaspoon garlic powder
- ¼ teaspoon cumin
- ¼ teaspoon salt
- ¼ teaspoon pepper
- ¼ teaspoon chili lime seasoning

HOW TO MAKE IT:

1. Mix garlic powder, cumin, salt, and pepper in a small bowl and set aside.
2. Combine corn, black beans, bell peppers, onion, mushroom, jalapeño, and lime juice in a bowl and mix well.
3. Lay chicken breasts flat in a large casserole dish and sprinkle evenly with seasoning.
4. Spread the vegetable mixture evenly over the chicken.
5. Top with shredded cheese.
6. Bake uncovered at 375°F for 40-50 minutes, or until chicken reaches an internal temperature of 160°F.
7. If cheese browns too quickly, loosely cover with foil for the remainder of cooking.
8. Serve warm.

NUTRITION (Per serving)

Calories: ~370
Protein: ~41 g
Total Carbohydrates: ~32 g
Dietary Fiber: ~9 g
Sugars: ~7 g
Total Fat: ~9 g
Saturated Fat: ~4 g
Sodium: ~525 mg

Chicken Primavera Spaghetti Squash Boats

This dish takes a classic pasta-style meal and lightens it up without losing the comfort factor. The spaghetti squash keeps things fresh and filling, while the chicken and vegetables bring real substance to the plate. It's a great option when you want something warm and satisfying that still feels aligned with how you're training and eating.

Serving Size: 4 servings

INGREDIENTS

- 12 oz cooked, shredded chicken breast
- 1 medium spaghetti squash, halved, seeds removed
- 1 tbsp extra-virgin olive oil
- ½ small red onion, chopped
- 1 orange bell pepper, chopped
- 1 tomato, chopped
- 1 medium zucchini, cut into half moons
- 2 cloves garlic, minced
- 1 tsp lemon zest
- Kosher salt
- Freshly ground black pepper
- ½ tsp Italian seasoning
- ½ cup shredded cheese
- ¼ cup freshly grated Parmesan

Freshly chopped parsley, for garnish

HOW TO MAKE IT (Instant Pot):

1. Carefully cut the spaghetti squash in half lengthwise and scoop out the seeds.
2. Pour 1 cup water into the Instant Pot and place the trivet inside.

3. Place squash halves on the trivet. Secure the lid, set the valve to Sealing, and cook on High Pressure for 7 minutes.
4. Perform a quick release, remove squash, let cool slightly, then shred the flesh with a fork. Leave strands in the shells to form "boats."
5. In a large skillet over medium heat, heat olive oil. Add onion and bell pepper and cook 3-4 minutes, until mostly tender.
6. Add tomato, zucchini, garlic, lemon zest, salt, pepper, and Italian seasoning. Cook 3-4 minutes more.
7. Stir in shredded chicken and remove from heat.
8. Divide chicken and vegetable mixture evenly between spaghetti squash boats and gently mix with strands.
9. Top each boat with shredded cheese.
10. Transfer to the oven and bake at 400°F for 5 minutes, until the cheese is melted.
11. Remove from the oven, sprinkle with Parmesan and parsley, and serve warm.

NUTRITION (Per serving)

Calories: ~394
Protein: ~37.0 g
Total Carbohydrates: ~20.6 g
Dietary Fiber: ~4.7 g
Sugars: ~5.4 g
Total Fat: ~13.5 g
Saturated Fat: ~4.7 g
Sodium: ~475 mg

Chicken Vegetable Casserole

This is a classic comfort dish cleaned up for everyday life. It's creamy without being heavy, balanced enough to feel like a real meal, and easy to portion for multiple days. When you want something familiar that still supports your goals, this casserole quietly gets the job done.

Serving Size: 6 servings

INGREDIENTS

- 12 oz cooked chicken breast, diced
- 7 oz whole wheat penne pasta
- 2 tablespoons unsalted butter
- 2 tablespoons all-purpose flour
- 10 oz skim milk
- 1 teaspoon Italian seasoning
- Pinch white pepper
- 1 tablespoon grated Parmesan cheese
- 2 yellow or orange bell peppers, chopped
- 1 zucchini, chopped
- 12 oz broccoli, chopped
- ⅓ cup Monterey Jack cheese
- Nonstick cooking spray

HOW TO MAKE IT

1. Preheat the oven to 350°F. Lightly coat a 9 × 13 baking dish with nonstick cooking spray.
2. Cook pasta according to package directions. During the final minute of cooking, add broccoli to the boiling water. Drain and set aside.
3. In a small saucepan over medium heat, melt butter. Add flour and stir continuously for 1 minute, avoiding browning.

4. Slowly add milk while whisking. Bring mixture to a gentle bubble, then reduce heat and simmer for 10 minutes until thickened.
5. Stir in Italian seasoning, white pepper, and Parmesan cheese.
6. In a large bowl, combine cooked pasta, broccoli, chicken, bell peppers, zucchini, and sauce. Mix gently.
7. Transfer mixture to prepared baking dish and sprinkle Monterey Jack cheese evenly over the top.
8. Cover with foil and bake for 20 minutes.
9. Remove foil and continue baking until cheese is fully melted.
10. Remove from the oven and serve warm.

NUTRITION (Per serving)

Calories: ~480
Protein: ~37.6 g
Total Carbohydrates: ~49.7 g
Dietary Fiber: ~8.4 g
Sugars: ~7.1 g
Total Fat: ~13.3 g
Saturated Fat: ~5.6 g
Sodium: ~345 mg

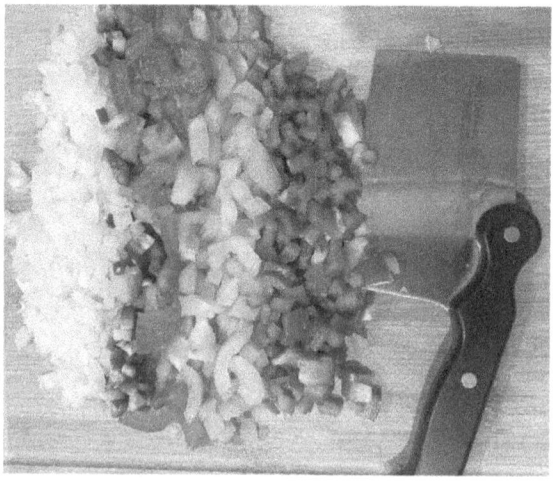

Creamy Spinach Spaghetti Squash Casserole

This is comfort food with a lighter footprint. The spaghetti squash keeps the dish filling without weighing you down, while the spinach and chicken add volume and protein where it counts. It's the kind of meal that feels indulgent but still fits cleanly into a consistent routine.

Serving Size: 4 servings

INGREDIENTS

- 12 oz chicken breast, diced
- 1 (3-pound) spaghetti squash
- ½ cup water
- 1 teaspoon olive oil
- 4 cups spinach, chopped
- ½ red bell pepper, diced
- 1 clove garlic, minced
- Dash of nutmeg
- 1 teaspoon salt
- ½ teaspoon pepper
- 5 oz cream cheese, softened
- 1 cup mozzarella cheese
- ¼ cup Parmesan cheese
- ¼ cup breadcrumbs

HOW TO MAKE IT (Instant Pot):

1. Carefully cut the spaghetti squash in half lengthwise and scoop out the seeds.
2. Pour ½ cup water into the Instant Pot and place the trivet inside.
3. Place squash halves on the trivet. Secure the lid, set the valve to Sealing, and cook on High Pressure for 7 minutes.

4. Perform a quick release, remove squash, let cool slightly, then shred into strands with a fork. Set aside.
5. Set Instant Pot to Sauté and add olive oil.
6. Add spinach and red bell pepper and sauté until spinach is wilted.
7. Add garlic, nutmeg, salt, and pepper and cook for about 1 minute, until fragrant.
8. Stir in cream cheese until melted and smooth.
9. Add shredded spaghetti squash and diced chicken. Stir gently to combine.
10. Lightly coat a casserole dish with cooking spray and transfer mixture into the dish.
11. Top with mozzarella, Parmesan, and breadcrumbs.
12. Bake at 375°F for 30 minutes, until bubbly and lightly browned.
13. Remove from the oven, let rest briefly, and serve warm.

NUTRITION (Per serving)

Calories: ~455
Protein: ~33.0 g
Total Carbohydrates: ~27.1 g
Dietary Fiber: ~5.1 g
Sugars: ~7.9 g
Total Fat: ~24.4 g
Saturated Fat: ~11.2 g
Sodium: ~1,063 mg

Honey Garlic Chicken - Instant Pot

This is a high-reward, low-effort dinner that delivers big flavor with almost no hands-on time. The Instant Pot keeps the chicken tender and juicy while the sweet-savory sauce makes it feel far more indulgent than it actually is. It's a great option when you want something comforting, fast, and easy to pair with rice or vegetables.

Serving Size: 4 servings

INGREDIENTS

- 1.5 pounds raw boneless skinless chicken breast
- 4 garlic cloves, minced
- ⅓ cup honey
- ½ cup low-sodium ketchup
- ½ cup low-sodium soy sauce
- ½ teaspoon dried oregano
- 2 tablespoons fresh parsley, chopped
- ½ tablespoon toasted sesame seeds

HOW TO MAKE IT (Instant Pot):

1. Place chicken breasts in the Instant Pot in a single layer.
2. In a bowl, whisk together garlic, honey, ketchup, soy sauce, oregano, and parsley.
3. Pour sauce evenly over the chicken.
4. Secure the lid, set the valve to Sealing, and cook on High Pressure for 10 minutes.
5. Allow a natural release for 5 minutes, then carefully perform a quick release.
6. Remove chicken and transfer to a serving plate.
7. Set Instant Pot to Sauté mode and simmer the sauce for 5-7 minutes, stirring occasionally, until slightly thickened.
8. Spoon sauce over the chicken.
9. Sprinkle the chicken with toasted sesame seeds and serve warm.

NUTRITION STATISTICS

Calories: ~380
Protein: ~49.5 g
Total Carbohydrates: ~29.5 g
Dietary Fiber: ~0.5 g
Sugars: ~23.0 g
Total Fat: ~5.5 g
Saturated Fat: ~1.1 g
Sodium: ~1,013 mg

Lemon Pepper Chicken - Instant Pot

This is a clean, protein-first staple designed for maximum flexibility. The lemon pepper keeps the flavor bright and simple, making it easy to pair with rice, quinoa, vegetables, or salads without getting repetitive. It's one of those "cook once, use everywhere" proteins that quietly supports consistency all week long.

Serving Size: 4 servings

INGREDIENTS

- 1 pound raw boneless skinless chicken breast, cut into strips
- 1 tablespoons olive oil
- 1 cup water (for Instant Pot)

Steve's Chicken Rub
(included in nutrition)

- 1 tablespoon lemon pepper
- 1 teaspoon sea salt
- 1 teaspoon garlic powder
- 1 teaspoon onion powder
- 1 teaspoon dried basil
- 1 teaspoon dried oregano
- 1 teaspoon dried parsley
- 1 teaspoon paprika

HOW TO MAKE IT (Instant Pot):

1. Season chicken breast strips generously with Steve's Chicken Rub.
2. Set Instant Pot to Sauté mode and add olive oil.
3. Season chicken breast strips generously with Steve's Chicken Rub.
4. Set Instant Pot to Sauté mode and add olive oil.
5. Lightly sear chicken strips until just golden.

6. Insert the trivet and add water to the bottom of the pot.
7. Place chicken on the trivet.
8. Secure the lid, set the valve to Sealing, and cook on High Pressure for 7-10 minutes.
9. Use a quick release or short natural release.
10. Remove chicken and serve immediately.

NUTRITION STATISTICS

Calories: ~195
Protein: ~31 g
Total Fat: ~7 g
Saturated Fat: ~1.5 g
Total Carbohydrates: ~1 g
Dietary Fiber: 0 g
Sugars: 0 g
Sodium: ~600 mg

OPTIONAL VARIATIONS

Turkey tenderloins instead of chicken. Your favorite lean beef cut. Just don't use my chicken rub on beef. Beef rubs exist for a reason — they're spectacular.

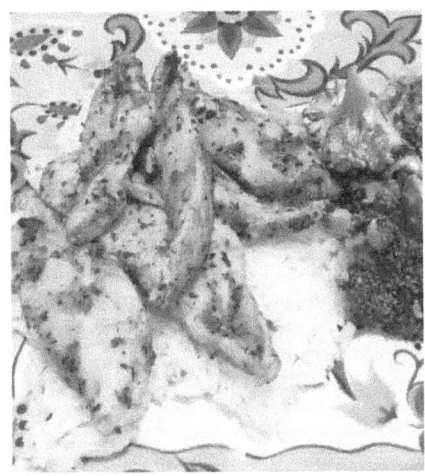

Mexican Cauliflower Rice Casserole

This dish delivers bold, comforting flavors in a lighter, vegetable-forward format. It works equally well as a standout side or as a complete meal when you add the optional protein boost. When you're training harder or just want volume without heaviness, this one earns its place.

Serving Size: 4 servings

INGREDIENTS

- Pinch of cayenne pepper
- 1½ teaspoons salt
- 1 (26.5 oz) can no-salt-added chopped tomatoes
- 1 pound cauliflower rice
- 3 large eggs, beaten
- 3 ounces reduced-fat Colby Jack cheese
- 1 tablespoon olive oil
- 1 medium onion, chopped
- 1 bell pepper, chopped
- 1 jalapeño, diced (seeds and white pith removed)
- 1 clove garlic, minced
- 1 teaspoon ground cumin
- 1 teaspoon chili powder

HOW TO MAKE IT:

1. Preheat the oven to 350°F.
2. Heat olive oil in a deep oven-safe skillet or Dutch oven over medium heat.
3. Add onion, bell pepper, and jalapeño. Sauté until tender, about 8–10 minutes.
4. Add garlic, cumin, chili powder, cayenne, and salt. Cook for 1 minute until fragrant.

5. Stir in chopped tomatoes and cauliflower rice. Once the mixture begins to simmer, lower heat, cover, and cook until vegetables are tender, about 8-10 minutes.
6. Remove from heat, uncover, and let cool slightly. Stir well.
7. Add beaten eggs and mix thoroughly to distribute evenly.
8. Top with reduced-fat Colby Jack cheese.
9. Bake at 350°F for 30 minutes, until eggs are set and cheese is bubbly and lightly golden.
10. Let rest 10 minutes before serving.

NUTRITION STATISTICS

Calories: ~230
Protein: ~13.0 g
Total Carbohydrates: ~17.0 g
Dietary Fiber: ~5.5 g
Sugars: ~6.5 g
Total Fat: ~13.0 g
Saturated Fat: ~4.0 g
Sodium: ~255 mg

Mexican Chicken and Cauliflower Rice Casserole

The base version of this dish makes an incredible side alongside a main protein. But when you're training harder, lifting heavier, or deliberately pushing toward a leaner body composition, this upgraded version lets the casserole stand on its own as the main event.

Adding shredded chicken doesn't change the soul of the recipe — it simply gives it more horsepower. Same flavors. Same simplicity. Just more protein and more staying power This is the meal I choose when I need more than just a full plate.

Serving Size: 4 servings

INGREDIENTS — PROTEIN BOOST ADD-ON

- 12 ounces cooked, shredded chicken breast
  (Season lightly with cumin, chili powder, garlic, and salt)

HOW TO MAKE IT (Protein Boost)

1. Prepare the Mexican Cauliflower Rice Casserole base as written.
2. Cook and shred the chicken breast separately. Season lightly with Mexican-style spices.
3. Before baking, fold the shredded chicken evenly into the casserole mixture.
4. Top with cheese as directed and bake according to the original recipe instructions.
5. Let rest briefly, then serve.

NUTRITION STATISTICS

   Calories: ~375
   Protein: ~36.0 g
   Total Carbohydrates: ~17.0 g
   Dietary Fiber: ~5.5 g
   Sugars: ~6.5 g
   Total Fat: ~14.5 g
   Saturated Fat: ~4.1 g
   Sodium: ~288 mg

Orange Chicken - Air Fryer

This is a takeout-style favorite rebuilt with a protein-first mindset and none of the usual baggage. You still get bold citrus flavor and that satisfying glaze, but in a version that feels light, clean, and energizing instead of heavy. It's fast enough for weeknights and familiar enough to feel like comfort food without the regret.

Serving Size: 2 servings

INGREDIENTS

- pound boneless skinless chicken breasts
- 2 tablespoons cornstarch or potato starch
- ½ cup orange juice
- 2 tablespoons brown sugar
- 1 tablespoon soy sauce
- 1 tablespoon rice wine vinegar
- ½ teaspoon freshly grated ginger
- Dash of red pepper flakes
- Zest of one orange
- 2 teaspoons cornstarch mixed with 2 teaspoons water
- Green onions, chopped
- Sesame seeds

HOW TO MAKE IT:

1. Preheat the air fryer to 400 degrees.
2. Combine chicken pieces and cornstarch into a bowl and mix until chicken is just fully coated.
3. Cook chicken for 7-9 minutes, shaking the basket halfway through, or until chicken reaches 165 degrees internally.
4. Meanwhile, combine orange juice, brown sugar, rice wine vinegar, soy sauce, ginger, red pepper flakes, and orange zest in a small saucepan over medium heat.

5. Bring mixture to a simmer and cook for 5 minutes.
6. Mix cornstarch and water together in a small bowl and add it to the orange sauce.
7. Let simmer for one additional minute while stirring, then remove from heat.
8. Remove chicken from the air fryer and combine with sauce.
9. Top with green onions and sesame seeds if desired and serve immediately.

NUTRITION STATISTICS

Calories: ~400
Protein: ~52 g
Total Carbohydrates: ~31 g
Dietary Fiber: ~0.5 g
Sugars: ~19 g
Total Fat: ~6.0 g
Saturated Fat: ~2 g
Sodium: ~457 mg

Pork Carnitas - Instant Pot

This set-it-and-forget-it protein delivers big flavor with little effort. The Instant Pot does the heavy lifting, giving you tender, versatile pork that works in bowls, wraps, or alongside vegetables. It's great for cooking sessions to fuel several meals without getting bored.

Serving Size: 10 servings

INGREDIENTS

- 1 (4.0 lb) lean boneless pork roast, cut into 2-inch chunks, excess fat trimmed
- Fine sea salt
- Freshly cracked black pepper
- 1 tablespoon olive oil

For the sauce

- 1 cup low-sodium chicken stock
- 1 head garlic, cloves separated, peeled, and minced
- ½ cup fresh orange juice
- ¼ cup fresh lime juice
- 1 teaspoon dried oregano
- 1 teaspoon ground cumin
- 1 teaspoon fine sea salt
- ½ teaspoon freshly cracked black pepper

HOW TO MAKE IT (Instant Pot):

1. In a medium bowl, whisk together all mojo sauce ingredients. Set aside.
2. Season pork chunks generously with salt and pepper.
3. Set Instant Pot to Sauté mode and add olive oil.

4. Working in batches, sear pork on all sides until browned. Transfer browned pork to a plate and repeat until all pork is seared. Turn off Sauté mode.
5. Return all pork to the Instant Pot and pour mojo sauce over the meat. Toss briefly to combine.
6. Secure the lid, set the valve to Sealing, and cook on High Pressure for 30 minutes.
7. Allow a natural release for 15 minutes, then carefully release remaining pressure.
8. Remove the lid and shred pork using two forks.
9. Preheat the oven broiler to high. Transfer shredded pork to a large baking sheet using a slotted spoon.
10. Spoon about one-third of the cooking juices over the pork and toss gently.
11. Broil for 4–5 minutes until the edges begin to crisp. Remove, spoon half of remaining juices over pork, toss, and broil for another 4–5 minutes.
12. Remove from the oven, spoon remaining juices over pork, toss gently, and serve warm

NUTRITION (per serving)

Calories: ~352

Protein: ~30.4 g

Total Carbohydrates: ~5.8 g

Dietary Fiber: ~0.3 g

Sugars: ~3.6 g

Total Fat: ~21.6 g

Saturated Fat: ~7.6 g

Sodium: ~325 mg

Pot Roast and Potatoes - Instant Pot

This is a classic, no-frills dinner that delivers comfort, satiety, and leftovers you'll actually look forward to. The Instant Pot turns a traditionally long cook into a practical weeknight option while keeping the meat tender and flavorful. It's a great reminder that hearty, traditional meals can still fit into a smart, structured approach.

Serving Size: 8 servings

INGREDIENTS

- 3 lb beef chuck roast, fully thawed
- 1 tablespoon olive oil
- 1 teaspoon salt
- 1 teaspoon onion powder
- 1 teaspoon garlic powder
- ½ teaspoon black pepper
- ½ teaspoon smoked paprika
- 1 lb baby red potatoes
- 4 large carrots, chopped
- 1 large yellow onion, chopped
- 4 cups low-sodium beef broth
- 2 tablespoons Worcestershire sauce

For the Gravy

- ¼ cup water
- 2 tablespoons cornstarch

HOW TO MAKE IT (Instant Pot):

1. Set Instant Pot to Sauté mode. In a small bowl, mix salt, onion powder, garlic powder, black pepper, and smoked paprika. Rub seasoning evenly over the roast.

2. Add olive oil to the pot. Sear the roast on all sides, about 3–4 minutes per side, until browned.
3. Cancel Sauté mode. Arrange potatoes, carrots, and onion around the roast.
4. Pour beef broth and Worcestershire sauce over everything.
5. Secure the lid, set the valve to Sealing, and cook on High Pressure for 60 minutes.
6. Allow a natural release for 10 minutes, then carefully release remaining pressure.
7. Transfer roast and vegetables to a serving platter. Shred roast into chunks.
8. Skim and discard visible fat from the cooking liquid.
9. Set Instant Pot to Soup or Sauté mode. Whisk water and cornstarch together, then stir into the hot liquid until gravy thickens.
10. Serve gravy over roast and vegetables.

NUTRITION STATISTICS

Calories: ~403
Protein: ~30.8 g
Total Carbohydrates: ~18.8 g
Dietary Fiber: ~2.6 g
Sugars: ~2.8 g
Total Fat: ~20.0 g
Saturated Fat: ~7.3 g
Sodium: ~431 mg

Salmon & Veggie Bake

This is a simple, no-drama dinner that delivers high-quality protein and healthy fats in one pan. Everything roasts together, which keeps cleanup easy and flavors clean and straightforward. It's ideal for nights when you want something nourishing that doesn't feel complicated.

Serving Size: 1 serving

INGREDIENTS

- 1 farm-raised Atlantic salmon fillet (8 oz, raw)
- ¼ cup broccoli
- ¼ cup asparagus
- ¼ cup cherry tomatoes
- ½ medium Honeycrisp apple, diced
- 2 tablespoons olive oil
- 1 teaspoon salt
- 1 teaspoon black pepper
- Trader Joe's Salmon Rub

HOW TO MAKE IT

1. Preheat the oven to 400°F.
2. Line a baking sheet with foil or parchment paper.
3. Place salmon on the baking sheet and season with salt, pepper, and Trader Joe's Salmon Rub.
4. Arrange broccoli, asparagus, cherry tomatoes, and diced apple around the salmon.
5. Drizzle olive oil evenly over the salmon and vegetables.
6. Bake for 18-22 minutes, depending on thickness, until salmon is cooked through and flakes easily.
7. Remove from the oven and serve immediately.

NUTRITION (per serving)

Calories: ~780
Protein: ~47 g
Total Carbohydrates: ~34 g
Dietary Fiber: ~8 g
Sugars: ~18 g
Total Fat: ~52 g
Saturated Fat: ~9 g
Sodium: ~1,550 mg

Sesame Chicken and Veggies — Sheet Pan

This is a fast, balanced dinner that delivers big flavor with minimal cleanup. Roasting everything together keeps the chicken juicy and the vegetables crisp, while the sesame-style sauce ties it all together without overwhelming the meal. It's a great option when you want something satisfying, familiar, and easy to portion.

Serving Size: 4 servings

INGREDIENTS

- 1 pound raw boneless skinless chicken breast, cut into 1-inch pieces
- 1 large head broccoli, chopped (about 2 cups)
- 8–10 asparagus spears
- 12 cherry tomatoes, halved
- 2 medium red bell peppers, cut into chunks
- 1 cup snap peas

The Sauce

- ¼ cup lower-sodium soy sauce
- 1 tablespoon sweet chili sauce
- 2 tablespoons honey
- 2 cloves garlic, minced
- 1 teaspoon fresh ginger, grated
- Salt and pepper, to taste

(Optional toppings: sesame seeds and green onions — excluded from nutrition)

HOW TO MAKE IT:

1. Preheat the oven to 400°F.
2. In a small saucepan, combine soy sauce, sweet chili sauce, honey, garlic, and ginger. Bring to a simmer over medium heat, whisking occasionally, until slightly thickened. Remove from heat.

3. Arrange chicken and vegetables on a sheet pan lightly coated with cooking spray. Season lightly with salt and pepper.
4. Drizzle half the sauce over the chicken and vegetables and toss to coat.
5. Bake for 20 minutes, tossing halfway through, until chicken is cooked through and vegetables are tender.
6. Drizzle remaining sauce over the top before serving.

NUTRITION STATISTICS

Calories: ~295
Protein: ~39.0 g
Total Carbohydrates: ~21.5 g
Dietary Fiber: ~4.5 g
Sugars: ~10.5 g
Total Fat: ~3.5 g
Saturated Fat: ~0.8 g
Sodium: ~880 mg

Shrimp Scampi

This is a simple, restaurant-style meal that comes together quickly and still feels special. The shrimp cook fast, the garlic and lemon keep everything bright, and it pairs easily with pasta, squash, or vegetables depending on your needs. When you want something lighter that still delivers flavor, this one hits the mark.

Serving Size: 4 servings

INGREDIENTS

- 1 pound raw shrimp, peeled and deveined
- 3 tablespoons butter
- 2 tablespoons olive oil
- 4 teaspoons garlic, minced
- 1 cup low-sodium chicken broth
- 1 teaspoon kosher salt
- ¼ teaspoon red pepper flakes
- Black pepper, to taste
- 3 tablespoons lemon juice
- Fresh parsley, chopped

HOW TO MAKE IT:

1. Heat a large skillet over medium heat. Add butter and olive oil and let it melt together.
2. Add garlic and sauté until fragrant, about 1 minute.
3. Pour in chicken broth, salt, red pepper flakes, and black pepper. Bring to a simmer and cook for about 2 minutes.
4. Add shrimp and cook until just pink and opaque, 2–4 minutes depending on size.
5. Stir in lemon juice and chopped parsley.
6. Remove from heat and serve immediately.

NUTRITION (per serving)

Calories: ~295
Protein: ~37 g
Total Carbohydrates: ~3 g
Dietary Fiber: ~0.3 g
Sugars: ~0.5 g
Total Fat: ~16 g
Saturated Fat: ~6 g
Sodium: ~488 mg

Spaghetti Squash with Ground Turkey and Marinara/Vodka Sauce - Instant Pot

This dish gives you all the comfort of a classic pasta night without the heavy aftermath. The spaghetti squash keeps things light, while the meat and vodka sauce bring richness and satisfaction where it counts. It's a great example of how you can keep familiar flavors and still stay aligned with your goals.

Serving Size: 8 servings

INGREDIENTS

- 1 spaghetti squash (about 3 lb)
- ½ cup water
- 1 pound 93% lean ground turkey
- 12 oz Carbone Vodka Sauce
- 12 oz Carbone Spaghetti Marinara Sauce
- 2 tablespoons Italian seasoning
- Salt and pepper, to taste

HOW TO MAKE IT (Instant Pot):

1. Cut spaghetti squash in half lengthwise and scoop out seeds.
2. Pour ½ cup water into the Instant Pot and insert the trivet.
3. Place squash halves on the trivet, cut side up.
4. Secure the lid, set the valve to Sealing, and cook on High Pressure for 7 minutes.
5. Quick release pressure and remove squash. Let cool slightly, then shred into strands with a fork.

Sauce and Protein

6. In a large pot over low-medium heat, combine marinara sauce, vodka sauce, and Italian seasoning. Warm gently.

7. In a separate pan, brown ground turkey over medium heat. Season lightly with salt and pepper.
8. Stir cooked turkey into the sauce mixture and heat through.

Assemble

9. Divide spaghetti squash strands among plates or a serving dish.
10. Spoon meat and sauce mixture over the squash and serve warm.

NUTRITION (per serving)

Calories: ~405
Protein: ~24.5 g
Total Carbohydrates: ~24.0 g
Dietary Fiber: ~3.5 g
Sugars: ~5.8 g
Total Fat: ~22.0 g
Saturated Fat: ~7.3 g
Sodium: ~606 mg

Spaghetti Squash with Ground Beef

Ground Turkey OR Ground Beef??

If you're like my Uncle and you just can't wrap your head around the thought of ground turkey…

Me: I need to run to the store for some ground turkey.

Uncle: Ground Turkey? You can't grind turkey meat!

Me: I am sure there was once a day when beef wasn't ground. I'm sure there were people then saying, "You can't grind beef!"

Uncle: Beef is the only thing that should be in a grinder!

Me: What about my weed?

Uncle: Huh?

Me: Nothing!

Anyway, this version gives you a richer, more classic comfort-food flavor while still keeping things intentional. Swapping in **93% lean ground beef** bumps the calories and saturated fat slightly, but it also delivers depth and familiarity that can make this dish feel more indulgent without going completely off the rails.

INGREDIENTS

- Swap 1 pound 93% lean ground turkey for 1 pound 93% lean ground beef

NUTRITION (per serving)

Calories: ~440
Protein: ~23.0 g
Total Carbohydrates: ~24.0 g
Dietary Fiber: ~3.5 g
Sugars: ~5.8 g
Total Fat: ~26.0 g
Saturated Fat: ~9.8 g
Sodium: ~612 mg

Note: This is an intentional swap, not a default. Use it when flavor, comfort, or family familiarity matters more than keeping saturated fat as low as possible.

Spaghetti Squash with Ground Chicken

If you want to keep the dish lighter while still changing up the protein, ground chicken is a great middle ground. It's lean, mild in flavor, and takes on the sauce beautifully without adding extra heaviness. Just don't tell my Uncle what you're doing! This version is ideal if you're:

- Prioritizing leanness but want something different than turkey
- Cooking for people who prefer a softer flavor
- Looking for variety without sacrificing momentum

It's familiar, flexible, and very easy to keep in regular rotation.

INGREDIENTS

- Swap 1 pound 93% lean ground turkey for 1 pound lean ground chicken

NUTRITION (per serving)

    Calories: ~390
    Protein: ~25.0 g
    Total Carbohydrates: ~24.0 g
    Dietary Fiber: ~3.5 g
    Sugars: ~5.8 g
    Total Fat: ~19.0 g
    Saturated Fat: ~5.8 g
    Sodium: ~600 mg

Why This Works:

Compared to turkey, ground chicken: Shaves off a bit of fat and calories, keeps protein strong and consistent, stays neutral enough to let the sauce lead.

Compared to beef, it's a clear step toward leanness while still feeling like a true comfort meal.

This is one of those swaps that makes long-term consistency easier — and that's always the real goal.

Spinach Stuffed Chicken Breasts

This is a protein-forward dinner that feels a little elevated without being complicated. The creamy spinach filling keeps the chicken moist and flavorful, while still fitting cleanly into a balanced plan. It's a great option when you want something that looks impressive but works just as well for meal prep.

Serving Size: 4 servings

INGREDIENTS

- 4 boneless skinless chicken breasts
- 1 tablespoon olive oil
- 1 teaspoon paprika
- 1 teaspoon salt, divided
- ¼ teaspoon garlic powder
- ¼ teaspoon onion powder

Spinach Filling

- 4 ounces reduced-fat cream cheese, softened
- ¼ cup grated Parmesan cheese
- 2 tablespoons light mayonnaise
- 1½ cups chopped fresh spinach
- 1 teaspoon garlic, minced
- ½ teaspoon red pepper flakes

HOW TO MAKE IT:

1. Preheat the oven to 375°F.
2. Place chicken breasts on a cutting board and drizzle lightly with olive oil.
3. In a small bowl, mix paprika, ½ teaspoon salt, garlic powder, and onion powder. Season both sides of the chicken.

4. Using a sharp knife, carefully cut a pocket into the side of each chicken breast.
5. In a bowl, mix cream cheese, Parmesan, light mayonnaise, spinach, garlic, red pepper flakes, and remaining ½ teaspoon salt until combined.
6. Spoon the spinach mixture evenly into each chicken breast.
7. Place stuffed chicken breasts in a 9 × 13 baking dish.
8. Bake uncovered for 25–30 minutes, until chicken is cooked through.
9. Remove from the oven and let rest briefly before serving.

NUTRITION STATISTICS

Calories: ~455
Protein: ~52.0 g
Total Carbohydrates: ~4.0 g
Dietary Fiber: ~1.0 g
Sugars: ~1.3 g
Total Fat: ~24.0 g
Saturated Fat: ~8.5 g
Sodium: ~875 mg

Stuffed Eggplant with Chicken

This is a hearty, satisfying dinner that leans on vegetables without feeling like a compromise. The eggplant becomes a sturdy base for a flavorful, protein-rich filling that eats like comfort food while still staying balanced. It's a great option when you want something different that still feels substantial and grounding.

Serving Size: 2 servings

INGREDIENTS

- 1 large eggplant
- 12 ounces extra-lean ground chicken
- 1 tablespoon extra-virgin olive oil
- ½ teaspoon grey sea salt
- ¼ teaspoon black pepper
- 1 onion, diced small (about 1 cup)
- 1 red bell pepper, diced small (about 1 cup)
- 3 cloves garlic, finely chopped
- 1 tomato, chopped
- ½ cup fresh parsley, chopped
- ½ cup fresh basil, chopped
- ¼ cup grated Parmesan cheese
- ¼ cup plain panko breadcrumbs
- 1 whole egg

HOW TO MAKE IT:

1. Preheat the oven to 350°F.
2. Slice the eggplant in half lengthwise and scoop out the center, leaving enough flesh to hold its shape. Chop the scooped eggplant.
3. Place chopped eggplant in a saucepan, cover with water, and boil until very soft, about 10–12 minutes. Drain well.

4. Heat olive oil in a sauté pan over medium heat. Add ground chicken, season with salt and pepper, and cook until lightly browned, breaking into small pieces.
5. In a separate pan, sauté onion, red bell pepper, and garlic until softened.
6. In a large bowl, combine cooked eggplant, chicken, sautéed vegetables, parsley, basil, Parmesan, panko, and egg. Mix until fully combined.
7. Fill the eggplant shells evenly with the mixture.
8. Top with chopped tomato.
9. Place in a lightly oiled baking dish and bake for 50 minutes.
10. Let cool briefly, slice widthwise, and serve.

NUTRITION STATISTICS

Calories: ~480
Protein: ~42 g
Total Carbohydrates: ~33 g
Dietary Fiber: ~8.5 g
Sugars: ~11.5 g
Total Fat: ~22 g
Saturated Fat: ~5.5 g
Sodium: ~825 mg

Thai Chicken Coconut Curry

This is a warm, comforting dinner that delivers bold flavor without relying on heaviness. The coconut curry sauce feels rich and satisfying, while the chicken and vegetables keep it balanced and nourishing. It's especially great when you want something cozy that still supports training, recovery, and consistency.

Serving Size: 6 servings

INGREDIENTS

- 1 pound boneless skinless chicken breast, diced
- 2 tablespoons coconut oil
- 1 medium/large yellow or Vidalia onion, diced
- 3 cloves garlic, minced
- 2 teaspoons ground ginger
- 1 (13 oz) can lite coconut milk
- About 3 cups fresh spinach
- 1 to 1½ cups shredded carrots
- 2 teaspoons ground coriander
- 2 tablespoons Thai red curry paste
- 1 teaspoon kosher salt
- ½ teaspoon freshly ground black pepper
- 1 tablespoon lime juice
- 1 tablespoon brown sugar
- ¼ cup fresh basil, chopped

HOW TO MAKE IT:

1. Heat coconut oil in a large skillet over medium-high heat.
2. Add onion and cook until softened, about 5 minutes.
3. Add chicken and cook until just cooked through, stirring often.
4. Stir in garlic, ginger, and coriander and cook until fragrant, about 1 minute.
5. Add coconut milk, carrots, curry paste, salt, pepper, and brown sugar. Stir well.
6. Reduce heat to medium and simmer gently for about 5 minutes, allowing flavors to develop.
7. Add spinach and stir until wilted, about 1–2 minutes.

8. Finish with lime juice and basil. Taste and adjust seasoning if needed.
9. Serve warm...over rice?

NUTRITION STATISTICS

Calories: ~347
Protein: ~25.0 g
Total Carbohydrates: ~13.0 g
Dietary Fiber: ~2.3 g
Sugars: ~3.7 g
Total Fat: ~19.7 g
Saturated Fat: ~12.0 g
Sodium: ~442 mg

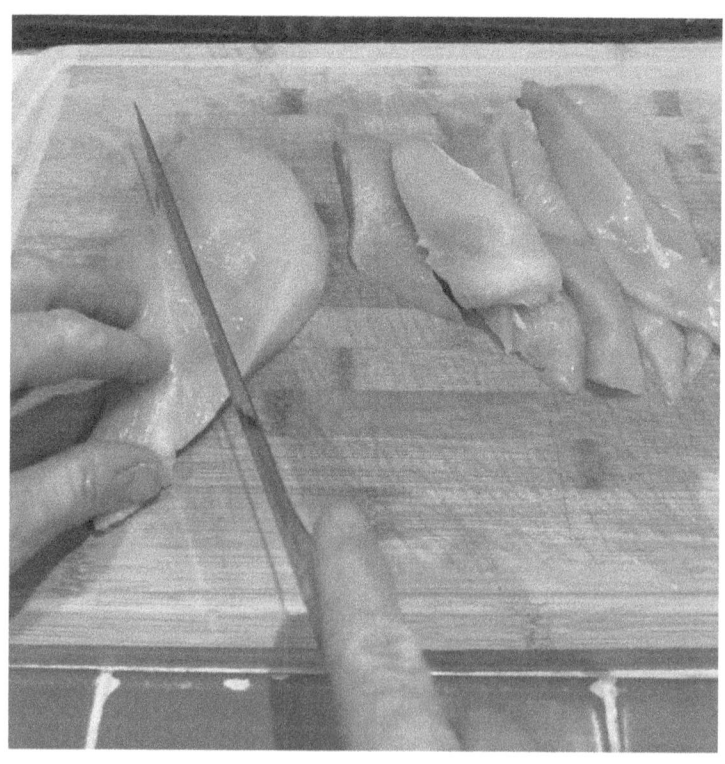

Thai Red Curry with Vegetables

This is a vibrant, vegetable-forward dish that brings big flavor and warmth without feeling heavy. It's flexible enough to stand on its own or pair easily with added protein, making it a smart choice on both lighter days and harder training days. When you want something bold, comforting, and still clean, this one fits perfectly.

Serving Size: 4 servings

INGREDIENTS

- 1 cup dry brown jasmine rice or long-grain brown rice
- 1 tablespoon coconut oil
- 1 small white onion, chopped (about 1 cup)
- Pinch of salt
- 1 tablespoon fresh ginger, finely grated
- 2 cloves garlic, minced
- 1 red bell pepper, sliced into thin strips
- 1 yellow, orange, or green bell pepper, sliced into thin strips
- ½ cup water
- 3 carrots, peeled and sliced (about 1 cup)
- 1½ cups thinly sliced kale (stems removed)
- 2 tablespoons Thai red curry paste
- 1 (14 oz) can lite coconut milk
- 1½ teaspoons coconut sugar or brown sugar
- 1½ tablespoons low-sodium tamari
- 2 teaspoons rice vinegar or fresh lime juice
- Fresh basil or cilantro, optional for garnish

HOW TO MAKE IT:

1. Cook brown rice according to package directions. Set aside.
2. Heat coconut oil in a large skillet over medium heat.
3. Add onion and a pinch of salt and cook until softened, about 5 minutes.
4. Stir in ginger and garlic and cook until fragrant, about 30 seconds.
5. Add bell peppers and carrots and cook until just tender, 3–5 minutes.
6. Stir in curry paste and cook for 1–2 minutes to bloom the spices.

7. Add coconut milk, water, kale, and sugar. Stir to combine.
8. Bring to a gentle simmer and cook for 5-10 minutes, until vegetables are tender.
9. Remove from heat and stir in tamari and rice vinegar or lime juice.
10. Serve curry over rice and garnish with fresh herbs if desired.

NUTRITION STATISTICS

Calories: ~340
Protein: ~9.0 g
Total Carbohydrates: ~48.0 g
Dietary Fiber: ~6.0 g
Sugars: ~7.0 g
Total Fat: ~13.0 g
Saturated Fat: ~8.5 g
Sodium: ~475 mg

Thai Red Curry with Vegetables + Shredded Chicken

If you love the flavors of this curry but want it to stand alone as a higher-protein meal, adding shredded chicken is an easy, clean upgrade. This version keeps the vegetable-forward feel while giving you the protein support you'll want on harder training days, heavier lifting cycles, or anytime dinner needs to pull more weight.

This is a perfect example of how meals evolve with momentum — same base, smarter fuel.

Serving Size: 4 servings

INGREDIENTS (Protein Boost Only)

- Add 12 ounces shredded chicken breast
 (prepared using the locked "Shredded Chicken (Instant Pot)" method)

(All other ingredients and instructions remain exactly the same as the base recipe.)

HOW TO MAKE IT (Protein Boost Adjustment):

- After the curry has simmered and vegetables are tender, fold in the shredded chicken.
- Stir gently and heat for 2-3 minutes until chicken is warmed through.
- Serve over rice as usual.

NUTRITION STATISTICS

Calories: ~425
Protein: ~27.0 g
Total Carbohydrates: ~48.0 g
Dietary Fiber: ~6.0 g
Sugars: ~7.0 g
Total Fat: ~14.0 g
Saturated Fat: ~8.5 g
Sodium: ~535 mg

Tilapia and Veggies

This is a clean, straightforward dinner that keeps things light, fast, and nutrient-dense. The mild tilapia pairs easily with roasted vegetables, making it a great option when you want protein without heaviness.

Serving Size: 2 servings

INGREDIENTS

- 12 ounces raw tilapia fillets
- 3 tablespoons butter, melted
- 2 cloves garlic, crushed and diced
- 2 cups broccoli florets (fresh or frozen)
- 1 large zucchini, sliced
- 1 cup baby carrots, halved
- 2 tablespoons lemon juice
- 3 teaspoons fresh parsley (or dried)
- 1 teaspoon oregano (fresh or dried)
- Salt and pepper, to taste

HOW TO MAKE IT:

1. Preheat the oven to 400°F.
2. In a small pan over low heat, melt butter. Add garlic and sauté gently for about 1 minute until fragrant. Remove from heat, stir in lemon juice, parsley, oregano, salt, and pepper.
3. Arrange tilapia fillets and vegetables in a single layer on a sheet pan.
4. Evenly pour the garlic butter mixture over the fish and vegetables.
5. Bake 12-15 minutes, until tilapia flakes easily, vegetables are tender.
6. Remove from the oven and serve immediately.

NUTRITION (per serving)

Calories: ~540
Protein: ~58.0 g
Total Carbohydrates: ~17 g
Dietary Fiber: ~5 g
Sugars: ~6.0 g
Total Fat: ~28.0 g
Saturated Fat: ~16.6 g
Sodium: ~310 mg

(Healthy) Tuna Noodle Casserole

This is a familiar classic rebuilt with smarter ingredients and better balance. It delivers comfort and nostalgia without the heaviness that usually comes with casseroles. When you want something warm, filling, and easy to portion for a few days, this one fits perfectly.

Serving Size: 4 servings

INGREDIENTS

- 2 (5 oz) cans water-packed tuna, drained
- 10 oz dry pasta shells (or rotini/fusilli)
- 3 tablespoons butter, divided
- 1 white onion, diced
- 8 oz baby bella mushrooms, sliced
- 1 teaspoon dried thyme
- Salt and pepper, to taste
- ¼ cup all-purpose flour
- 1¾ cups unsweetened almond milk
- ½ teaspoon garlic powder
- ½ cup reduced-fat grated Parmesan cheese
- 1 cup frozen peas

For the topping

- ½ cup breadcrumbs
- 1 tablespoon butter

HOW TO MAKE IT:

1. Preheat the oven to 350°F. Lightly coat a 9 × 9 baking dish with nonstick cooking spray.
2. Cook pasta according to package directions until al dente. Drain and set aside.
3. In a large skillet over medium heat, melt 1 tablespoon butter. Add onion, mushrooms, thyme, salt, and pepper. Cook for 4-6 minutes until vegetables are softened. Transfer to a bowl.
4. In the same skillet, melt remaining 2 tablespoons butter. Whisk in flour, then slowly add almond milk while whisking to avoid lumps. Bring to a gentle boil, then reduce heat and simmer until thickened.

5. Turn off heat and stir in garlic powder and Parmesan cheese.
6. Add cooked pasta, mushroom mixture, tuna, and peas to the sauce. Stir gently to combine and adjust seasoning if needed.
7. Transfer mixture to prepared baking dish.
8. In a small bowl, mix breadcrumbs with 1 tablespoon melted butter. Sprinkle evenly over the casserole.
9. Bake uncovered for 20-30 minutes, until bubbly and lightly golden on top.
10. Remove from the oven and let rest briefly before serving.

NUTRITION (per serving)

    Calories: ~495
    Protein: ~36.5 g
    Total Carbohydrates: ~58.0 g
    Dietary Fiber: ~4.5 g
    Sugars: ~5.0 g
    Total Fat: ~14.8 g
    Saturated Fat: ~6.8 g
    Sodium: ~455 mg

Wok Protein & Veggie Bowl

This is the ultimate "build once, eat all week" meal. It's efficient, satisfying, and one of the most reliable tools in the entire FF50 playbook.

Serving Size: 4 servings

INGREDIENTS - Vegetable Base

- 4-5 broccoli florets
- 4-5 cauliflower florets
- ½ carrot, sliced
- ½ green bell pepper, chopped
- ½ red bell pepper, chopped
- ½ zucchini, chopped
- 4 ounces mushrooms
- 4 ounces spinach
- ½ white onion, diced
- 1 medium jalapeño, finely chopped
- 1 tablespoon minced garlic
- 2 tablespoons olive oil
- 1 teaspoon sea salt
- 1 teaspoon Black Pepper

NUTRITION — BASE ONLY

Calories: ~290
Protein: ~10 g
Total Carbohydrates: ~24 g
Dietary Fiber: ~8 g
Sugars: ~7 g
Total Fat: ~20 g
Saturated Fat: ~3 g
Sodium: ~640 mg

Protein Options
Choose One — 1 pound

- Lean ground turkey (93%)
- Lean ground beef (93%)
- Lean ground chicken
- Shrimp

HOW TO MAKE IT:

1. Heat a wok over medium heat and add olive oil before the pan gets too hot.
2. Add vegetables by density: carrots and broccoli first, then cauliflower, peppers, zucchini, mushrooms, onion, and spinach.
3. Cook, stirring frequently, until vegetables soften and begin to caramelize slightly.
4. Add garlic and jalapeño and cook briefly until fragrant.
5. Season vegetables with salt and pepper.

6. In a separate pan, cook your chosen protein until fully done.
7. Fold cooked protein into the vegetables gently.
8. Serve immediately.

NUTRITION (per serving) — BASE +

    With Lean Ground Turkey

        Calories: ~440

        Protein: ~36 g

        Total Fat: ~27 g

        Saturated Fat: ~5 g

        Sodium: ~720 mg

    With Lean Ground Beef (93%)

        Calories: ~480

        Protein: ~34 g

        Total Fat: ~32 g

        Saturated Fat: ~9 g

        Sodium: ~730 mg

    With Lean Ground Chicken

        Calories: ~410

        Protein: ~39 g

        Total Fat: ~23 g

        Saturated Fat: ~4 g

        Sodium: ~705 mg

    With Shrimp

        Calories: ~360

        Protein: ~37 g

        Total Fat: ~21 g

        Saturated Fat: ~3.5 g

        Sodium: ~850 mg

ESTEBAN'S GUAC FOR THE WOK

Use it wherever, and whenever you want!

Serving Size: 2 tablespoons, Makes 8 servings

INGREDIENTS

- 2 large avocados (or 3 medium)
- Juice of ½ lime
- Juice of ½ lemon
- ½ teaspoon sea salt
- Red onion, finely diced
- Fresh cilantro, chopped
- Jalapeño, finely diced

HOW TO MAKE IT:

- Check Avocado ripeness. I read somewhere that they should be about as hard as the thumb muscle inside your palm. I hope that helps you too!
- In a small dish, mix the onion, cilantro, jalapeño, and citrus juice, set aside.
- Slice open Avocados, remove pits.
- Scoop into a mixing bowl.
- Mash with salt.
- Add the "small dish" mixture into the mashed avocado and fold gently.

NUTRITION STATISTICS

Calories: ~60
Protein: ~1 g
Total Carbohydrates: ~3 g
Dietary Fiber: ~2 g
Sugars: ~0.5 g
Total Fat: ~5 g
Saturated Fat: ~0.8 g
Sodium: ~75 mg

PART III — The Shift
Where identity turns action into a way of life

CHAPTER NINE
Mindset: The Identity Shift

At some point during this process, something strange happened. Not dramatic. Not cinematic. No "rocky montage" moment where the music swells and the camera circles. I didn't wake up one day feeling motivated. I didn't suddenly love discipline. I didn't even feel especially proud. What I felt was… calm.

Calm in the way you feel when you stop arguing with yourself.

Calm in the way you feel when the decision has already been made.

Calm in the way you feel when you're no longer asking, *"Should I?"*

That's the part most people miss.

We're trained to look for change to feel loud. Emotional. Transformational. We expect fireworks. A before-and-after picture with arrows and captions. We expect effort to announce itself. But the thing that actually made this work didn't show up like that at all.

It Showed Up As Silence.

The noise disappeared. The internal debate. The daily negotiation. The running commentary of *"I'll start tomorrow"* versus *"I deserve this today."* That voice didn't get louder. It retired. And in its place was something much less exciting and far more powerful: alignment.

I wasn't forcing new behavior. I wasn't borrowing discipline from the future. I wasn't dragging guilt from the past. I was simply acting in a way that matched who I had already decided to be. That's the shift. Not trying harder. Not wanting it more. Not proving anything to anyone. Just protecting an identity that finally felt settled.

Most people think success is about adding something—more rules, more motivation, more structure. What actually happened here was the opposite. Things were removed. Permission was gone. Negotiation was gone. Decision fatigue was gone. And when those things disappeared, consistency didn't feel heroic. It felt obvious.

This chapter isn't about what I did. You already know that. You've seen the meals, the systems, the plans, the microstrategies that stacked up over time. This chapter is about *why those things finally worked*. Because for the first time, I wasn't trying to become someone new. I was protecting someone I already was.

For most of my life, this wasn't even a conversation. I was active. Athletic. Functional. My body worked the way it always had. I didn't bounce between diet plans or workout programs trying to fix a problem. I worked out because that's what I did. I moved because movement was normal.

The weight didn't arrive with an announcement. It showed up quietly. A comfortable relationship. Great meals. Date nights that revolved around restaurants. A flying career built on airport food, odd hours, and convenience. Nothing reckless. Nothing dramatic. Just a slow reverse compound effect doing exactly what compound effects do.

By the time I noticed, it wasn't because everything had gone wrong. It was because alignment had drifted. And that's why this process mattered so much. This wasn't about "trying again." There was no pattern to repeat or program to restart. This was the first time I had to deliberately take ownership of something that had changed without asking me first.

That's where a lesson from a fire captain resurfaced—not as a story, but as a standard. Years ago, he taught me something simple: *your name is on this*. If something went wrong, your name was attached to it. If something went right, your name was attached to that too. There was no hiding behind effort. No partial credit for intention. Your name either carried weight—or it didn't.

For a long time, my health lived in a gray area. Not neglected. Not prioritized. Just assumed. This time, I put my name on it. And when your name is on something, you don't negotiate with it the same way. You don't ask how little you can get away with. You don't wait to see how things unfold. You step up.

That's where discipline gets misunderstood. Discipline isn't force. It isn't punishment. It isn't white-knuckling through discomfort. When it's working, discipline is simply refusing to act in a way that embarrasses the version of you you've already committed to being. Discipline is self-respect.

And self-respect doesn't yell. It doesn't bargain. It isn't threatening. It quietly says, *"That's not how we do things anymore."*

Once that standard was set, preparation stopped feeling obsessive and started feeling obvious. It wasn't about control. It was about protection. You protect what matters. You prepare for what carries your name.

Once my name was on it, something else shifted that I didn't immediately notice. The way I talked to myself changed. Not in a motivational way. Not affirmations. Not hype. The language tightened.

Years ago, Pat Alexander drilled a principle into me that stuck because it worked: **language becomes instruction**. The words you use don't just describe what you're doing. They tell you what to do next.

For a long time, my internal language was loose. Casual. Harmless-sounding. *I'll clean this up. I'll be better this week. I'll get back on track.* None of that sounded irresponsible. But none of it gave clear direction either.

Once I committed—once my name was on it—vague language stopped working. Because vague language creates vague behavior. So the words changed. Not louder. Shorter.

Instead of *"I'll try to stay on track,"* it became: *This is what I eat.*

Instead of *"I should work out more consistently,"* it became: *This is when I train.*

Instead of *"I'll be good during the week,"* it became: *This is how I operate.*

Those aren't motivational phrases. They're operational ones. They remove emotion. They remove debate. They remove the need to decide in the moment. Once language became instructional, behavior didn't need to be forced. It followed.

That's when my internal voice changed. For years, it wasn't cruel—but it wasn't helpful either. It commented on everything. It kept score. It analyzed outcomes after the fact. That's what critics do. A critic shows up after the moment has passed and tells you how you should've handled it.

A coach shows up before the moment—and tells you what to do next.

Once my language tightened, the critic retired. The voice in my head stopped narrating my performance and started guiding it. *Eat this. Train now. Go to bed.* No tone. No judgment. No story attached.

At first, it felt almost cold. But it wasn't cold. It was respectful. The critic assumes you need to be convinced. The coach assumes you're already committed. And once you're committed, commentary becomes unnecessary. This is where people get stuck. They think they need more motivation, when what they actually need is less commentary. Because commentary invites emotion. Emotion invites negotiation. Negotiation invites drift. A coach eliminates all three.

And when your internal voice becomes a strength coach, you don't feel controlled. You feel supported.

The final shift sealed everything. Permission disappeared. Permission sounds harmless. Reasonable, even. *Do I get to today? Have I earned this? Can I let this slide just once?* But permission is a loophole disguised as kindness. Choice is different. Choice is clean. Choice doesn't ask how the day's going. Choice doesn't require justification. Choice closes the conversation.

I didn't deny myself anything. I didn't forbid foods. I didn't restrict my life. I simply stopped asking for permission. Because permission implies you might say yes. Choice implies you already decided. Once that line was crossed, willpower became irrelevant. There was nothing to resist. Nothing to white-knuckle. Nothing to stay strong against. The decision had already been made by the version of me I trusted.

When I look back now, it's obvious why this worked. Putting my name on it established the identity. Tightening my language turned that identity into instruction. Replacing permission with choice removed negotiation entirely.

Once those three aligned, nothing else needed to be forced. Preparation became protection, not control. Discipline became self-respect, not effort. Consistency stopped being something I managed and started being something I maintained.

I wasn't trying to change anymore. I was protecting who I'd already become.

CHAPTER TEN
Microstrategies That Shaped My Journey

There are certain chapters in a book that are about mindset and philosophy. There are chapters about results and identity. This chapter is different.

This chapter is about survival. This is the chapter you come back to when the day goes sideways, when your schedule collapses, when you didn't prep, when you didn't get to the store, when life happened and now you're standing in your kitchen asking yourself, *"Okay... now what?"*

There will be imperfect days. These are not heroic efforts. These are the small moves that shaped my journey. The microstrategies that helped navigate through the noise. Quiet decisions that didn't look impressive in the moment but compounded over time and kept me moving forward. This chapter isn't about being flawless. It's about staying in the game.

Microstrategy 1: Empowering Your Will

Everybody talks about willpower, the importance of having willpower. I would like to say something important about willpower. I don't see willpower as an enemy to be overcome. I understand it as the empowerment of your will. Once you start tasting these meals—once you realize how delicious they are—you don't have to worry so much about what they're doing to your body on the inside. That work happens quietly, behind the scenes.

So really, this is about having the power of your will to try new things. The power to cook in your own kitchen. The power to use an Instant Pot for the first time. When you champion the power of your will, your boundaries expand. And once your mind expands, it never goes back.

Microstrategy 2: Hydration Situation

The cleanse teaches you something most people never learn: hydration is not optional, and it's not cosmetic. The cleanse will teach you to drink a lot of distilled water. The cleanse will show you that you can have over a gallon of water a day and your body will actually appreciate it. Energy improves. Clarity improves. Hunger becomes quieter. You feel steady.

Then the cleanse ends and the real question shows up. After the cleanse, what do you drink then? The obvious answer is nature's elixir, water. But if not water, I knew it had to be zero sugar. I originally started my zero sugar journey with a well-known sports drink, the one named after the football team at the University of Florida, whose name rhymes with Haterade. When I was drinking that particular zero sugar sports drink, my ankles started to swell. Not from injury, just barely puffy. It had never happened to me before.

My mom, being a nurse, asked a simple question. How much salt are you taking in? I said the regular amount. The only change in my diet was the extra sports drinks. Then I looked at the label. 170 milligrams of sodium per serving. I was absolutely shocked.

I looked around and I found Vitamin Water. Zero sugar, zero sodium, multiple flavors, sarcastic comments on the bottle! I immediately made the switch and never went back. The swelling disappeared. Thank you, Vitamin Water. Thank you, 50 Cent.

Microstrategy 3: Never Get Hangry

Hungry is normal. Hangry is different.
 Hungry is human. Hangry is a human condition.

Hangry is when hunger turns into a mood. When you stop thinking clearly. When the voice shows up that says, "Just get something, anything, and get it now."

Most breakdowns in the system are not the cause of food. They are the cause of timing. It starts from waiting too long. It starts from thinking you can power through without fuel. That's like asking your car to continue to drive when the empty light turned on thirty miles ago.

Hydration helps, timing your snacks helps, and proper prep helps. But the rule itself is simple and non-negotiable.

Never get hangry.

Microstrategy 4: Mini-Losses Don't Matter — Repetition Does

A mini-loss is when you fail to prep or fail to get to the store. It will happen. You are human.

When it happens, don't beat yourself up. Accept it. Order the pizza. Enjoy the pizza. Then get right back into your system as soon as possible. Not Monday. Not next week. Next meal.

No one expects perfection. Only progress. When we fail, we restart.

This also applies to splurges. Go to the Super Bowl party. Have eighteen wings, four beers, and three slices of pizza. Enjoy your birthday cake. Dig in on Thanksgiving. You have earned it. Congratulate yourself for earning a day off—not a cheat day.

The term cheat day is poor psychology. Reward beats shame every time.

Microstrategy 5: Grocery Ordering Is Energy Protection

I absolutely love ordering through Amazon Fresh or Whole Foods Delivery. If I know I'm going to have a busy day, I can have what I need delivered. I don't worry about spending four or five dollars on delivery. I worry about spending forty-five to ninety minutes in a store making bad decisions.

Unfortunately, you can't always trust someone else to know what a good avocado feels like, what a ripe cantaloupe smells like, or the difference between a green banana and a yellow banana. I know it sounds simple, but you'd be shocked at what I've received.

It's not a joke when I say I've gotten avocados as hard as baseballs. They looked like oversized limes and took a full week to ripen — uh, excuse me, I'm trying to have guacamole tonight.

So while ordering is great for dry goods, spices, and meat, I prefer to be hands-on when selecting my fruits and vegetables.

Swap the proteins. Have fun with the substitutions. Shrimp one day, fish the next. This isn't laziness — this is strategy. Be creative. I live mostly in the chicken, fish, and shrimp world, this way I can say "yes" to a delicious burger.

Microstrategy 6: Prep Today for Tomorrow

Prep isn't becoming a different person. Prep is about protecting future you from the chaos. Prep is about learning what you need before you need it.

As you went through the first three weeks, as you go through the first three weeks of learning in your kitchen before the cleanse, you also learn about prep and creating grocery lists and those lists covering three days' worth of food to eliminate daily trips to the store. Being prepared also creates flexibility.

This isn't glamorous. It's strategic. Tomorrow doesn't get to ambush you when tonight already did the work.

Another cheat code when it comes to prep—especially if you're single— is understanding portion reality. Sometimes you can cut the recipes in half. Other times you can't. When I make a full recipe, I eat my meal, then immediately cut the rest into portions, put them in glass containers, and stick them in the freezer.

Microstrategy 7: Freeze, Seal, and Deploy

In the last Microstrategy, you might have thought it was a typo when I said to put leftovers in the freezer. Let's be clear. I don't leave food sitting loosely in the freezer, because freezer burn is real. The move is simple but specific: freeze the food first, then seal it properly so it's protected, preserved, and ready when you need it.

This system comes from my years as a flight attendant. When I was trying to eat better while constantly on the road, this was the procedure. Make a meal. Split it into portions. Freeze them. Seal them in FoodSaver bags. Because the meals were frozen solid, I could pack two of them into my food bag and take them with me. One meal per night. No stress. No scrambling.

I'd finish flying, get to the hotel, change into my gym clothes, and put a frozen meal into my HotLogic. By the time I got back from the gym, dinner was ready. Many people aren't familiar with what a HotLogic is, but it's simple: it gently heats your food over time. We'll include a link, because once you use one, it's hard to go back.

Most of this book isn't about saving time — it's about maximizing it. The beauty of this system is that when you cook a few nights in a row and eat something different each time, you suddenly have extra portions. When you freeze and seal them properly, they can last for weeks without freezer burn.

That's when this becomes powerful. You build a grab-and-go, whatever-you-feel-like-eating system. You put a frozen meal into your HotLogic, walk away like it's a load of laundry, and go live your life for thirty-five or forty minutes.

I know that might sound counterintuitive in a book that praises the Instant Pot and air fryer for speed. But this is about compounding effort. You cook once, and future dinners take care of themselves. You come back, open the container, and you're eating like a king.

Microstrategy 8: Confidence Expands Your World

I have never seen a more green steamed broccoli than the first time I opened the Instant Pot. Rice that comes out fluffy every time. An unlimited way of making beef and chicken. To go from forty minutes in a traditional oven to make a spaghetti squash down to just over seven minutes is absolutely ridiculous. I cannot give the Instant Pot enough praise.

Because of its flexibility, I feel like I can cook virtually anything with the Instant Pot. Last Christmas, I even found an Instant Pot recipe for tamales, and they were delicious.

The Instant Pot isn't all about speed. It's about confidence. It's about looking at a recipe and saying, "I can do this." Every kitchen appliance you learn removes friction and resistance. Every win expands your boundaries and your beliefs. And like the saying says, once your mind expands, it can never go back.

Microstrategy 9: Spice, Spice, Baby

Learning how to cook involves learning how to work with spices.

No one expects you to take a list of spices from this book and go buy all of them at once. But hey, if you're fired up and you're feeling it… do it. Do it.

For the rest of you, start small. Start with the first five basics. Slowly add a couple at a time. Over time, you'll build an incredible spice rack.

Part of me wanted to list the top five or the top ten spices here. But that would only be *my* top five or *my* top ten. Anyone can do a Google search and find the most popular spices. What matters more is experience. I recommend going through the first three weeks using the spices that show up naturally during that time. By the time you come out of the cleanse, you're almost a spice master without even realizing it.

And more important than having the spice rack is having the knowledge and understanding of how to use it.

We'll provide a link to an easy-to-create, easy-to-grow spice rack.

Microstrategy 10: Shredded Chicken — The Ultimate Cheat Code

Shredded chicken is one of the foundations that holds everything together. It's flexible, reliable, and quietly powerful. It can become whatever the day needs it to be. When plans change, shredded chicken removes friction instead of adding stress.

Being able to make shredded chicken quickly in an Instant Pot has been a game-changer. In minutes, you have protein ready to go. It turns vegetables into meals, snacks into fuel, and side dishes into something substantial.

Shredded Chicken (Instant Pot)

How to Make It

1. Place chicken breasts in the Instant Pot in a single layer.
2. Add 1 cup water or low-sodium chicken broth to the pot.
3. Season lightly with salt and pepper if desired.
4. Secure the lid and set the valve to Sealing.
5. Cook on High Pressure for 10 minutes.
6. Allow a natural release for 5 minutes, then carefully perform a quick release.
7. Remove chicken and shred with two forks.

When protein is already made, decisions get easier. And when decisions get easier, consistency becomes possible.

Microstrategy 11: The Elephant in the Kitchen

I'm going to talk about the elephant in the kitchen now. And that is the microwave. I don't like it. I don't believe in it. And I won't use it.

Three reasons.

Number one: I personally feel there's a connection between the evolution of microwaved and heavily processed foods and the massive epidemic of unhealthy, disease-prone human beings in the United States.

Number two: I believe there's an unfortunate connection between the profits of the processed food industry and the health industry. Profits not only from eating the food, but from dealing with the long-term effects of eating that food. This isn't a book about the health industry, but I do know I don't want to support systems that profit from bad food leading to bad outcomes.

Number three: I don't like the taste. Plain and simple. Food doesn't taste the same when it's microwaved. Bread reminds me of Big League Chew from Little League—without the great flavor. I fully believe as you read this, you know exactly what I'm talking about.

It might take a little extra time to load up the air fryer or drop a teaspoon of olive oil into the same pan or wok you cooked in the night before and warm food slowly, thoroughly, and properly. But food tastes like food again.

Standup comedian Brian Regan has a great joke about how ridiculous it is that there are microwave directions on a Pop-Tart box. You're instructed to *"Microwave it for three seconds."* It's upsetting that we can't find thirty to forty-five seconds to properly toast a "Fruit"-filled pastry.
   "How do I get that goodness in me?" — Brian Regan

Microstrategy 12: Fast-Food Pivots (Survival Without Shame)

When it comes to fast food, I have a massive weakness for Southern California In-N-Out Burger. And when I say massive weakness, I mean it. I went there nearly every day through my late twenties and thirties. I even have a tattoo of the Los Angeles skyline on the inside of my right forearm, and down at the bottom of that skyline is a small restaurant with crisscross palm trees. This is how much I love In-N-Out Burger.

After the cleanse, I felt empowered enough to return to my love for In-N-Out—but differently. Their famous burger is a Double-Double. I prefer a Double-Single. Half the cheese calories, day after day, week after week. That compound effect matters. I also get it with no sauce. My grandma told me to try it that way, and it was life-changing. You still get the animal-style mustard flavor without the calorie-packed dressing.

When I'm in a workout phase, I'll take it further and order protein style, which is basically a lettuce wrap. I've referenced this throughout the book as a way to cheat bread calories. The same goes elsewhere. If you're at Subway, order the six-inch and rip off the top bread. Eat it open-faced. Looks weird. Sounds weird. Your body will thank you.

If you're getting tacos, get the tacos—but choose guacamole over sour cream. Better fats, same creamy satisfaction. These aren't sacrifices. These are pivots. Fast-food survival without shame. You don't need perfection. You need options.

If there's one thing I hope this chapter made clear, it's this: none of this requires heroics. No white-knuckling. No personality transplant. No becoming "that guy" who won't stop talking about macros at a dinner party. These are microstrategies. Small moves. Quiet decisions. The kind that don't get applause but absolutely get results.

The first part of this chapter was about stabilizing the inside. Empowering your will. Drinking enough water. Eating before you turn into a completely different human being. And maybe most importantly, letting go of the idea that one imperfect moment somehow invalidates everything you've done. Hunger, dehydration, and shame are a dangerous trio. When those are handled, you're already ahead of the game.

Next it was all about protecting your energy. Or maybe more accurately, becoming aware of how easily your energy gets drained. Most bad food decisions aren't made because you're lazy. They're made because you're tired, rushed, overwhelmed, or standing in a grocery store aisle negotiating with a version of yourself who hasn't eaten in six hours. Ordering groceries, prepping ahead, freezing meals—none of that is about discipline. It's about removing unnecessary friction and setting traps for your future self. Good traps.

Then, the conversation moved to confidence. Learning tools. Learning flavors. Building a few reliable foundations that quietly hold everything together. Confidence doesn't come from knowing everything. It comes from knowing enough. Enough spices to make food taste good. Enough appliances to make cooking feel possible. Enough shredded chicken in the fridge so dinner doesn't turn into a philosophical debate. As confidence increases, stress decreases.

And finally, we talked about how all of this fits into real life. Drawing a line where it matters—like how you heat your food—while staying flexible where life demands it. You don't win by avoiding fast food forever. You win by knowing how to pivot when it shows up. Half the cheese. No sauce. Lettuce wrap. Guacamole instead of sour cream. You're not cheating the system. You're navigating it.

This system works because it doesn't ask you to be perfect. It asks you to stay in the game. To recover faster. To think one step ahead. To build systems that work even when motivation doesn't show up.

These microstrategies didn't change my life overnight. They changed my life quietly, over time, while I wasn't looking. And that's usually how the best changes happen.

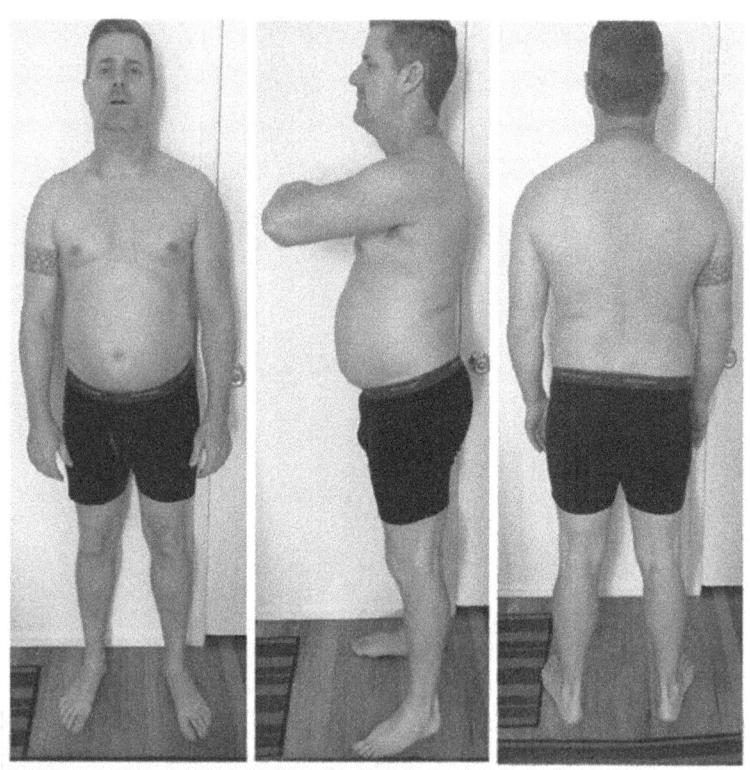

I didn't recognize the drift while it was happening.

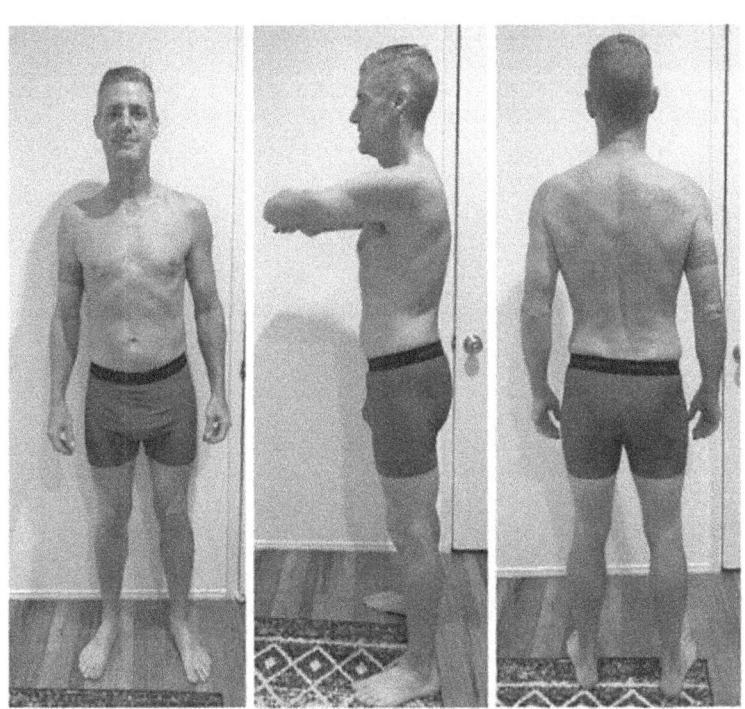

I recognized myself again.

CHAPTER ELEVEN
The Results: Fit and Flexible at 50

This isn't a victory lap. It's a receipt.

Results were never the point of this process. They were the byproduct. The goal was alignment—between how I ate, how I moved, how I prepared, and how I thought. The results simply showed up once those pieces stopped fighting each other. Still, a fair question remains: *Did this actually work?*

That's what this chapter is for.

Not to sell you on anything. There's nothing to sell. Not to hype a transformation. There's nothing to hype. Just to show you what changed—physically, mentally, and emotionally—when I stopped trying to fix my body and started building a system I could live inside.

What follows isn't dramatic. There are no shortcuts, no heroics, no secrets. Just facts, patterns, and honest observations from the other side of consistency. Take what's useful. Ignore what isn't. This isn't about copying my path. It's about seeing what's possible when preparation replaces willpower.

The Numbers (The Facts)

I'm putting the numbers first for a simple reason: they answer the practical question before the emotional one.

I started at **206 pounds**.

I finished at **156 pounds**.

Total loss of **50 pounds**.

My waist went from **36+ inches to 31 inches**.

I went back to my high school waistline. Where are my old Shrink-to-Fit, Levi 501s?

All my clothes fit differently. Shirts hang instead of pulling. Pants don't require negotiation. Belts moved inward, notch by notch, without ceremony.

About halfway through the process, I realized something else was happening: I was going to need a new wardrobe. By the end, that turned out to be very true. Large became medium. Medium became small. Pants either needed to be hemmed or replaced entirely. It wasn't dramatic—it was just logistics catching up with the data.

There were no gimmicks involved. No tricks. No extreme measures. No "one weird thing." I didn't starve. I didn't suffer. I didn't chase speed. The numbers changed because the inputs changed—and then stayed changed long enough to matter.

That's all the data you need. The rest of this chapter is about what those numbers don't show.

The Feeling (What Changed Internally)

The most meaningful changes didn't show up on a scale or a tape measure.

Energy came back first—not the jittery kind, not the short-term motivation surge, but a steady, reliable energy that carried through the day. Mornings stopped feeling like recovery sessions, and getting out of bed didn't require negotiations with my joints.

Movement became easier. Not impressive. Just easier. I noticed it in small moments: bending down without thinking about it, getting up from a chair without bracing, walking without stiffness tagging along for the first ten minutes.

Flexibility returned quietly. It wasn't something I trained aggressively. It was something that reappeared once inflammation dropped and daily movement became normal again.

Confidence changed too, but not in a loud way. There was no urge to prove anything. It felt more like being comfortable taking up my own space again—physically and mentally. I felt at home in my body, which is a subtle thing until you've been without it.

One of the most unexpected changes was sleep. My body started running so efficiently that I simply didn't need more than about six hours. Not because of insomnia, and not because I was wired or restless. I would wake up because my body was ready to go. My brain felt alert. My system felt online.

That changed my mornings completely. 5:30 a.m. became normal. Then 5:00 a.m. became normal. And this wasn't coming from going to bed at seven o'clock like an old man trying to win a sleep contest. I was still enjoying my evenings. I was still going to bed at eleven or even midnight. But after six hours, my body was done resting.

What that unlocked was time. Real time. I could finish a yoga workout and eat breakfast before 7:00 a.m.—at an hour when I used to just be waking up. Mornings stopped being something I survived and started being something I used.

Flexibility showed up the same way—quietly, without drama. I used to watch yoga videos and assume the people on screen were operating with some inhuman level of mobility that simply wasn't available to me. Over time, without forcing it, I found myself needing a yoga block for deeper stretches. Not to show off. Not to "achieve" anything. Just because my body could now access ranges of motion it couldn't before.

All the things golfers try to grind their way toward on the range started improving as a side effect of being lighter, looser, and more mobile. I didn't practice more. I didn't train harder. I just moved better. That might be the most important lesson I've learned through this entire process.

The impact on my golf game was undeniable.

Bigger rotation

Longer drives.

More consistent irons.

The weight loss was the headline result—fifty pounds gone—but the side effects were the real gift. And they didn't disappear once the scale stopped moving. They're still here.

There was also the simple, human change of recognizing my own face again. The jawline I remembered came back. The extra fullness disappeared. It wasn't about vanity as much as familiarity—seeing myself in the mirror and feeling like the image matched how I felt inside.

Looking back, the biggest wins weren't visible in the mirror. They showed up in how often my body felt like an ally instead of a project.

What Didn't Change

Despite everything that changed, a lot stayed exactly the same.

I still eat enjoyable food. Meals are satisfying, familiar, and flexible. Nothing about this required turning eating into a performance or a math problem.

I'm still human. I have off days. I miss workouts. I eat things that weren't "planned." None of that broke the system.

There was no obsession. No constant tracking. No weighing myself every morning. No anxiety around social events or travel. Food didn't become something I had to control—it became something I worked with.

I didn't chase perfection. I didn't need it. Consistency handled what willpower never could.

This process didn't shrink my life to make room for results. It fit inside the life I was already living. That's an important distinction, because results that require restriction eventually require rebellion. This didn't.

One unexpected byproduct of this process showed up in a place no one writes about—but everyone understands.

As my body became more efficient, everything slowed down in a good way. Food was processed properly. Nutrients were absorbed instead of rushed through. I actually ate less, not because I was restricting, but because my body retained more of what it was given.

And then there was digestion. For years, like most people, going to the bathroom meant cleanup. You wipe, you check, you wipe again. That was just normal.

Then, somewhere along the way, something changed. I wiped—and there was nothing there. I assumed I'd missed. I folded the paper and tried again. Still nothing. It was genuinely confusing.

The only comparison I could come up with was this: my poops were suddenly as clean as a dog's. Nothing to clean up. No residue. No aftermath.

It sounds ridiculous, but it was also unmistakable evidence. The machine was running flawlessly.

The Identity Shift Made Visible

Somewhere along the way, the work stopped feeling like effort and started feeling like identity.

I became someone who prepares. Meals weren't decided in moments of hunger—they were decided ahead of time, calmly, when I had perspective. That single shift removed more friction than any rule ever could.

I became someone who moves daily. Not in a heroic way. Not with punishment or performance attached. Movement became a baseline expectation, like brushing my teeth or going for a walk. It happened because that's what I do now.

I became someone who protects energy. I stopped borrowing against tomorrow with late nights, poor food choices, and skipped movement. Decisions started running through a simple filter: *Does this support how I want to feel tomorrow?*

And maybe most importantly, I became someone who trusts themselves. I stopped negotiating with my own intentions. When I said I'd prepare, I prepared. When I said I'd move, I moved. That trust compounded quietly over time.

None of this required a personality change. It didn't demand discipline upgrades or motivational speeches. It was the natural outcome of aligning systems with values—something this book has been building toward since the very beginning. What changed wasn't just my body. It was the relationship I had with it.

The Compound Effect

Nothing about this process was dramatic.

There were no single days that changed everything. No breakthrough workouts. No moments where I felt like I'd "turned a corner" overnight.

What worked was the accumulation of small choices, repeated long enough to matter.

Walking happened daily. Stretching happened regularly. Not because it was impressive, but because it was easy to return to. Movement wasn't intense—it was consistent.

Meals were chosen ahead of time. That eliminated decision fatigue and prevented small moments of hunger from turning into poor choices. I wasn't relying on restraint. I was relying on preparation.

As my execution in the kitchen improved, my confidence grew. As my confidence grew, my spice rack grew. And as my spice rack grew, so did my freedom.

I stopped living strictly inside recipes and started flowing between them—borrowing techniques, marrying concepts, and creating meals that were specific to what I actually enjoyed. Cooking stopped being about compliance and started being about expression.

That didn't happen all at once. It was another compound effect. Small skills stacking into confidence, confidence stacking into creativity, creativity making consistency easier instead of harder.

Microstrategies did most of the heavy lifting. Simple guardrails that prevented derailment before it started. Nothing rigid. Nothing heroic. Just enough structure to keep momentum intact.

And once momentum existed, motivation followed—not the other way around. I didn't wait to feel inspired to act. Action created the feeling that people usually chase first.

Looking back, the compound effect is almost boring to describe. That's part of the point. The results didn't come from doing anything extreme. They came from doing the ordinary things, repeatedly, without quitting.

Why This Is Sustainable

There was no finish line attached to this process.

I never framed it as a countdown or a temporary phase. There was no moment where I told myself, *Once I get there, I can stop.* That mindset is what makes most results fragile.

This wasn't a comeback story. It was a transition into maintenance.

The systems I built weren't designed to produce a dramatic "after." They were designed to be livable—on busy weeks, during travel, and in normal life. That's why they held.

Fit and flexible isn't something I achieved and moved past. It's a state I maintain. A way of operating that adjusts instead of breaks.

When there's no rush, there's no rebound. When there's no deprivation, there's nothing to revolt against. That's the difference between results that fade and results that stay.

Gratitude and Realism

I'm grateful for the results, but more than that, I'm grateful for the clarity. I'm grateful that I learned these lessons when I did—even if it took longer than I would've preferred. Late didn't turn out to be too late. It turned out to be right on time.

There's effort in this story, and I own that. I prepared. I showed up. I stayed consistent. But there's also luck—having access to good food, time to move, and the opportunity to pay attention before something forced me to.

This chapter isn't about claiming credit. It's about acknowledging reality. Progress usually comes from effort meeting opportunity, not from one or the other alone.

I don't feel superior for having done this. I feel grounded. Grateful to be moving better, thinking clearer, and living in a body that feels cooperative again.

That's enough.

As I Reflect

The results didn't make me worthy. They didn't give me discipline, character, or value. All of that was already there. The work just stripped away the noise that had been hiding it.

This process didn't give me a new body. It gave me my body back.

Fit and flexible at fifty isn't about age. It's about alignment—between what you do, how you think, and what you're willing to sustain.

The numbers mattered. The feelings mattered more. But neither of them matters as much as knowing this is repeatable, livable, and real.

That's the result that lasts.

CHAPTER TWELVE
Now It's Your Turn

We've talked a lot about mentors in this book. Some were mentors to me before I ever knew they were mentors. One of my more recent mentors, Mr. Jim Rohn, said:

"Don't let learning lead to knowledge. Let learning lead to action."

This is not the end of the book. It's the handoff. It's where knowledge turns into action.

If you're here, you didn't skim. You didn't dabble. You stayed with it. And that matters more than you probably realize. Most people never make it this far—not because they can't, but because they stop trusting themselves halfway through. You didn't.

If you're feeling a little uncertain right now, that's normal. If part of you is excited and another part of you is hesitant, that's normal too. If you're waiting to feel "ready," that's normal—and unnecessary.

You don't need confidence to begin. You don't need clarity. You don't even need belief. You just need a starting point. And you already have one.

You Don't Need My Journey

You don't need my schedule, my meals, my routines, my timeline, or my exact results.

Your body is different. Your history is different. Your responsibilities are different. Your age, your work, your stress, your sleep—none of it matches mine, and it's not supposed to.

This was never meant to be a formula. It's a framework.

A lot of books like this will give you a defined 90-day meal plan. Every time I see one of those, it feels constricting and rigid. I prefer to give you the freedom to build your own based on your likes, your tastes, your schedule, your body, your life.

Take what fits. Adjust what doesn't. Leave the rest behind without guilt or explanation. The goal was never imitation—it was alignment. Alignment with how you actually live, how you actually move, and how you actually make decisions.

When your choices match your life, progress becomes sustainable.

Start Where You Are

There is no perfect Monday coming. There is no clean slate required. There is no moment where everything resets at once.

You don't need to overhaul your life. One meal prepared ahead of time counts. One walk counts. One stretch counts. One better grocery decision counts.

Momentum rarely announces itself. Most of the time, it starts quietly—small enough that people underestimate it and skip it entirely. The smallest action done consistently will outpace the grand plan that never starts.

Start where you are. Not where you think you should be.

What Actually Matters

If there's anything worth carrying forward, it's this: preparation beats motivation, identity outlasts willpower, consistency matters more than intensity, and progress wins over perfection.

None of that requires talent. None of it requires discipline as a personality trait. It requires choosing a few things that matter and doing them often enough that they stop feeling dramatic.

You don't need to do more. You need to do fewer things more reliably.

You Are Not Broken

You can't drive a car staring into the rearview mirror. It's there for reference, not direction. Looking back occasionally can be useful, but living there guarantees you never fully arrive anywhere new.

Whatever didn't work before doesn't disqualify you now.

The past is not a forecast. It's a record—and records can be learned from without being relived. Self-trust isn't something you either have or don't have. It's something you rebuild through small promises kept to yourself.

This time can be different. Not because you're a different person, but because you're approaching it differently. With more awareness. With less punishment. With a longer view.

You're not starting over. You're starting informed.

The Next Right Move

Here's the only question that matters right now: what is the next thing you can do today that makes tomorrow easier?

That answer won't be dramatic. It will probably feel almost too simple. That's a good sign.

Lower the bar on purpose. Make the win obvious. Prepare something small that future-you will quietly appreciate. That's how momentum is built—by making the right choice easier before you need it.

My Invitation To You

Fit and Flexible isn't a finish line. It's a formula of moving through life, with patience instead of pressure, with curiosity instead of judgment, and with consistency instead of intensity.

You don't need to prove anything. You don't need to measure yourself against anyone else. You don't need to get it right the first time. You're allowed to begin. And you're allowed to begin imperfectly.

That's not a weakness. That's empowering your will.

I have a sign over my front door. As I leave, I read it. It says:

"Don't look back. You're not going that way."

EPILOGUE

Five Years Later: Life at 55

The proof isn't what changed. It's what stayed.

Five years isn't dramatic. It's quiet. Enough time passes that no one is watching anymore. No one is tracking your progress. No one is asking how it's going. The applause is long gone, if there ever was any. What's left is just life—and how you live inside it.

So this isn't an update report. It's not a victory lap. It's a reflection on what happened after the goal stopped mattering.

The real test wasn't losing the weight. It was living after.

What Stayed the Same

I still prepare most of my meals.

Not perfectly. Not obsessively. But consistently enough that my body knows what to expect. I still walk. I still stretch. I still prioritize flexibility over force. I still choose movement that fits into my life instead of trying to bend my life around movement.

I'm still flexible instead of rigid. Still human. Still capable of overdoing things—and still capable of noticing sooner.

Most importantly, I'm still choosing alignment over extremes.

The habits didn't disappear when the goal did. They simply stopped needing to be announced.

What Changed—Subtly

About a year into this journey, I got excited. Too excited.

I had hit my one-year anniversary, felt incredible, and decided to celebrate by doing another seven-day cleanse. Five days in, I was already down nine pounds. And that's when something quietly clicked.

It took forty-nine years to build a body that needed a cleanse. It took one year of eating differently to convince me I didn't. That realization mattered more than the weight loss ever did.

I wasn't broken anymore. I wasn't correcting the damage. I was maintaining alignment. The system didn't need drama. It needed trust.

Since then, there's been less tracking and more intuition. Less urgency and more listening. Food became fuel again—and enjoyment—without negotiation or guilt. Movement became maintenance, not transformation.

Life didn't get smaller. It got fuller. The system evolved. It didn't break.

What Didn't Happen

I didn't rebound. I didn't need another reset. I didn't chase new programs. I didn't spiral when life got busy. And life did get busy.

What surprised me most is that none of this required vigilance. It required identity. Once I stopped treating my body like a project and started treating it like a partnership, there was nothing left to police.

Fit and Flexible didn't demand attention anymore. It just stayed.

Where I Am Now

At my lightest, I reached 156 pounds. At five-foot-eleven, that wasn't something I wanted—or needed—to sustain. I've always felt my best around 165 to 170. Strong. Athletic. Nimble.

As I move past my fifty-fifth birthday and into the December 2025 holidays, my biometric scale says I weigh 171.5 pounds, 18% body fat, 78% muscle, with other water, bone, and BMI numbers scrolling across the screen I don't feel I need to completely understand.

What I do understand is this: For the last three years, I have been wearing 32" golf pants that fit perfectly. I'm still palms-to-the-ground flexible. Still using a yoga block for deep stretches. Still walking miles of golf while carrying my bag—no push cart. Still regularly outdriving players younger than me.

More importantly, my doctor says my health numbers look fantastic for a 40 year old!

This is as close to being in the best shape of my life—across the board—as I've ever been. Not because I'm chasing it. Because I'm living inside it.

I feel at home in my body. Emotionally. Physically. Spiritually.

The Real Win

The win was never the body. It was the energy to work and create. Patience in relationships. The quiet confidence that comes from not negotiating with yourself all day.

The freedom from guilt. The absence of drama. Fit and flexible became the background, not foreground. And that's the point.

A Message, Looking Back

If I could speak to myself at the beginning—or to you, right now—it wouldn't be urgent. I'd say this: You don't need to rush. You don't need to be perfect. You don't need to become someone else. You're not behind. You're not broken. You're learning how to live in a body you respect. That's enough.

This was never about weight. It was about trust. It was about alignment. It was about learning how to live—calmly, honestly, sustainably—inside your own skin. Nothing to prove. Nothing to chase.

Just a life at home that feels aligned.

Acknowledgments & Influences

No journey like this happens in a vacuum. While this book is rooted in my own lived experience, there are a few people and ideas that influenced how I thought, how I prepared, and ultimately how I changed. They deserve recognition.

My father, Richard Monroe, while helping a young man learn the life lessons required to grow into adulthood, never let go of his childhood spirit. He always maintained the ability to be a goofball, and he is very much a catalyst for why I eventually found my way into stand-up comedy. My father played four years of minor league baseball for the New York Yankees, and his connection to sports has always been an anchor to my athleticism. He was also the first person to teach me how to play golf. One of his favorite sayings has stayed with me my entire life: *"Kid, there are no strangers — there are just friends you haven't met yet."*

My mother, Joyce Fowlkes has been an unwavering supporter of creativity itself. I've heard it said that every creator needs a support system, and I can't imagine what it must have been like for her to raise not one, but two creative types. What I can say without hesitation is that she believed deeply in the skills and abilities of her kids long before there was any proof to point to. Her steady encouragement and belief gave both my sister and me the confidence to explore, commit to, and ultimately thrive in our respective creative outlets. "Don't quit 5 minutes before the miracle!"

My step-father, Luis Cardenes is one of the top 5 most influential people in my life. Ailed by complications of Type I childhood diabetes, Luis lost his eyesight before the age of 30. Numerous trips to and from the doctor's offices. Through it all, he never, ever complained. Fueled by a need to forge his own path, Luis was the first to show me the life of working for yourself and being an entrepreneur. Over the years that I worked for him, the depth of the stories we shared helped guide me to my journey into stand up comedy.

Coach Pat Alexander was one of the first adults outside my family to shape how I understood my own mind. As a high school study skills teacher and coach of multiple sports, he introduced me to the concept of positive mental attitude and the relationship between conscious thought and subconscious belief. Long before nutrition or fitness entered my life, those lessons planted the idea that the words we speak to ourselves quietly shape who we become. "If it is to be, it is up to me."

David Littleton was my high school English teacher, and his connection to me — and the rest of the class — came from a youthful spirit that made learning feel alive. I didn't just take standard English from him. I took college vocabulary, creative writing, and Shakespeare. Thirty-five years later, I'm still honored to call Dave Littleton a very close friend. He has always inspired and encouraged my creative writing and storytelling, and this book carries more of his influence than he probably realizes.

Dr. William Davis, through his book *Wheat Belly, Lose the Wheat, Lose the weight, and find your path back to health*, Dr. Davis challenged the way I thought about food, digestion, and visceral fat. While I don't quote his work directly in this book, the concepts I learned there influenced how I viewed grains, inflammation, and how modern eating patterns affect the body. More importantly, that book pushed me toward curiosity instead of blind habit — a theme that runs throughout this journey. Many of the FF50 recipes were inspired within those pages.

There were also meaningful conversations with people whose names I no longer remember but whose words have never faded. One of them was the inspirational Fire Captain I spoke with during this period of change. In a simple, grounded way, he reinforced the importance of preparation, routine, and respecting the body as a tool that needs care, not punishment. Sometimes wisdom arrives briefly, says what it needs to say, and moves on. His message of respecting your name is something I instill into the junior golfers I am blessed to coach.

Special thanks to my personal physician, Dr. Christine Szeto, my best friends Rodney Jarvela, Steve Vinyard, Mataya Olson, Jason Hollingshead, my DVD trainer Tony Horton, and especially the casting directors with the Wheel of Fortune. Thank you Pat Sajak, Vanna White, and even the WOF photographer.

Finally, I want to acknowledge the quieter influences — the routines, the repetitions, the small daily decisions. The grocery trips. The walks. The stretches. The meals are cooked at home. The consistency that doesn't photograph well but changes everything over time.

This book isn't built on one breakthrough moment or one perfect plan. It's built on learning, listening, and being willing to adjust. I'm grateful to everyone and everything that nudged me in that direction.

Good luck!

You got this!

ABOUT THE AUTHOR

Steve Monroe was born in Southern California and raised mostly in Washington State. After high school, he found his way back to Southern California for college and beyond.

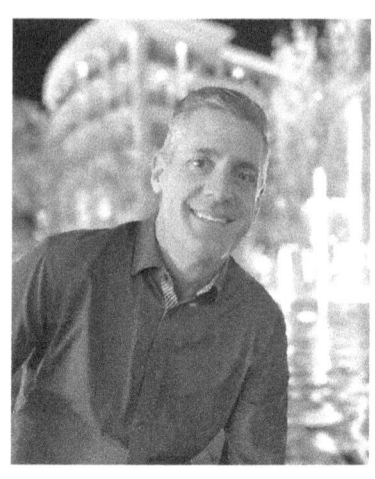

Curious by nature, Steve has always followed opportunity and experience, building a life that reflects becoming growth-minded, heart-centered, and committed to mastery. His career path has included bartending during college, working as a snowboard instructor, serving as a catering director, and getting fired from a corporate job for telling jokes. That firing led Steve to take a leap into stand-up comedy—a leap that turned into a career spanning more than two decades.

For most of his life, Steve was athletic and active, never someone who struggled with weight or movement. Over time, however—through career shifts, relationships, comfort, and the gradual realities of middle age—his body quietly changed. In his late forties, during the global pause of the pandemic, he reached a personal and physical turning point. What began as simple choices—eating clean, stretching daily, walking, playing golf, and paying attention—led to a complete shift in how he approached health and movement. The journey wasn't about extremes; it was about consistency, awareness, and rebuilding trust with his body.

That same mindset eventually led Steve into coaching. He returned to college and entered the PGA Management Program, quickly building a career in golf instruction, becoming a First Assistant Golf Professional and Director of Junior Golf. Teaching young people leadership and life skills through golf became one of the most meaningful chapters of his life.

Today, Steve is a Los Angeles based stand-up comedian, drone pilot instructor *@droneprola*, poet, and golf coach. He is also the author of the children's book *Penny and Noodle: Two Tails of Friendship*.

Fit and Flexible at 50 was written because friends, strangers, and personal experiences all pointed to the same truth: sustainable change matters most when it fits real life.

www.ingramcontent.com/pod-product-compliance
Lightning Source LLC
Chambersburg PA
CBHW061941130526
44582CB00040B/39